THE WARRIOR
AS HEALER

THE
WARRIOR
AS HEALER

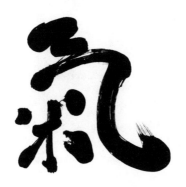

A MARTIAL ARTS HERBAL FOR
POWER, FITNESS, AND FOCUS

Thomas Richard Joiner

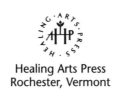

Healing Arts Press
Rochester, Vermont

Healing Arts Press
One Park Street
Rochester, Vermont 05767
www.InnerTraditions.com

Healing Arts Press is a division of Inner Traditions International

*Note to the reader: This book is intended as an informational guide. The remedies,
approaches, and techniques described herein are meant to supplement, and not to be
a substitute for, professional medical care or treatment. They should not be used to
treat a serious ailment without prior consultation with a qualified health care
professional.*

Library of Congress Cataloging-in-Publication Data
Joiner, Thomas Richard, 1943–
    The warrior as healer : a marital arts herbal for power, fitness, and focus /
Thomas Richard Joiner.
        p.   cm.
    ISBN 0-89281-796-8 (alk. paper)
    1. Herbs—Therapeutic use.   2. Martial arts injuries—Alternative
treatment.   3. Medicine, Chinese.   I. Title.
    RM666.H33J65 1999
    614'.321—dc21   99-27931
                                                                  CIP

Printed and bound in Canada

10 9 8 7 6 5 4 3 2 1

Text design and layout by Kristin Camp
This book was typeset in Caslon with Calligraphic as the display typeface

CONTENTS

ACKNOWLEDGMENTS

I would like to begin this first effort at book writing by expressing my heartfelt gratitude to some of the people who have taught and inspired me:

Master Mantak Chia of Taoist Esoteric Yoga, New York City; Urayoanna Trinidad of the Institute of Traditional Chinese Medicine/First World Acupuncture, New York City; Professor Lai Fu Chai of the Academy of Chinese Culture and Health Sciences, Oakland, California; and last but not least, my martial arts instructor and mentor, Shidoshi Ron Van Clief, Tenth-Degree Red Belt, Grandmaster of the Chinese Goju System, New York City.

I would also like to express my sincere thanks to Wu Shu-Chen for her beautiful calligraphy.

Author's Note

I strongly recommend that all martial artists, especially those on the teaching levels (*sensei* or *sifu*), become familiar with the basic first aid procedures practiced in Western medicine. The American Red Cross publishes an excellent book on these techniques, *Advanced First Aid and Emergency Care*. The herbal formulas that I present in chapter 2, "Injury-Management Formulas," can be used as an adjunct to the basic first-aid procedures described and taught by the American Red Cross.

The information in this book reflects current therapeutic knowledge. The self-treatment recommendations and information are appropriate in most cases; however, they are not a substitute for medical diagnosis. For specific information concerning your personal medical condition, you should consult a physician. Remember that you use any of the information offered within this book at your own risk. I cannot be held responsible for the results of any self-treatment you attempt on the basis of anything you read in this book.

The names of organizations, products, or alternative therapies appearing in this book are given for informational purposes only. Their inclusion does not imply endorsement; nor does the omission of any organization, product, or alternative therapy indicate disapproval.

PREFACE

early a quarter of a century has passed since the martial arts first became popular in the United States, in the early 1970s. Since then, escalating crime and violence have caused a steady increase in the number of people who are studying martial arts in an effort to acquire basic self-defense skills. It is estimated that as many as eight to ten million Americans are currently studying some form of martial arts.

Although the information that I present in this book can be useful to anyone on any level of training, it will likely have the greatest appeal to those martial artists who are committed to adopting the philosophical and spiritual tenets of traditional martial arts, rather than those whose interest is limited to basic self-defense training.

I wrote this book with two goals in mind: to inspire you to consider joining the new breed of martial artists who recognize the importance of reestablishing the historical relationship between the healing arts and martial arts; and to encourage you to learn how to use and incorporate Chinese herbs in your martial arts training. If you do so, the savage nature of combat—although not totally reconciled—will be diminished as a result of the increased level of human compassion you develop by integrating the two arts. In addition, the benefits of herbal use for improving your overall health and athletic performance will become obvious to you.

Literature that chronicles the use of herbs by martial artists date back many thousands of years. A number of books have been published that catalog herbal formulas used by martial artists for enhancing external (physical) training as well as internal (psychic) training. Other formulas developed by the grandmasters of martial arts systems remain secret and unpublished: their use is limited to members of a particular school or training system.

Although many ancient herbal formulas that were mainly used in martial arts have found their way into the mainstream of traditional Chinese medicine, there remains a number of manuscripts containing herbal formulas used by martial artists that have never been translated into English. Consequently, little is known about them. Still, although information identifying individual herbs and instruction in the use of formulas is somewhat scarce—at least when compared with the amount of available material that describes combat or fighting technique—I did find the following publications useful while researching this book: *Chinese Medicine in Injury Management; Chinese Herbal Medicine Materia Medica; Chinese Herbal Patent Formulas; Shaolin and Taoist Herbal Formulas;* and *Secret Formula for the Treatment of External Injury.* (For bibliographic information on these books, see appendix 5.)

What I must admit, however, is that in each case, although these books were scholarly and well written, all too often their information on martial arts philosophy (which was based on Eastern philosophical concepts) was obscured by cultural differences. In addition, the use of their herbal formulas was made difficult by botanical references in Latin and unnecessarily complicated medical language.

What I have attempted to do in this book, then, is combine the philosophy and history of martial arts with the use of Chinese herbs in an informal way that is not only factual but also easily readable. The formulas I discuss range from basic tonics that will increase *chi* (which, according to Chinese medical definition, is the vital energy or life force present in all living things) to preparations used to enhance meditation. Also included are some of the more exotic prescriptions that nourish the sexual reproductive energies—what traditional Chinese medicine refers to as *jing* essence.

These latter formulas are useful in the Taoist practice of sexual conservation, which is based on the pronouncements of the seventh-century physician Liu Ching. His ideas concerning the relationship between regulated sex, health, and longevity are incorporated in the practice known as Liu Fang Ching. This practice is said to hold the key to transmutation of the sexual energy, which is considered the purest form of energy (beyond even nutrition) and is perhaps one of the few remaining and most highly guarded secrets of esoteric martial arts.

I present the formulas in two basic forms: the raw form, which is fresh herbs that must be prepared from scratch, and patent formulas that are commercially prepared and packaged, usually as pills, tablets, capsules, liniments, syrups, and salves.

While patent formulas are generally easier and more convenient to use, I find that using herbs in their raw form has certain aesthetic and technical advantages that I will discuss in chapter 1.

Obviously, my purpose for writing this book will not be realized unless you become familiar with the formulas that I present by using them. My deepest wish is that this book will appeal to martial artists, regardless of their style, on an intellectual as well as a practical level. I hope that it will not be just read with casual interest and forgotten, but learned, applied, and passed on, in the true martial arts tradition.

INTRODUCTION

What makes my story different from those of most martial artists is that my training began not during childhood but at age thirty-one. Under the tutelage of Shidoshi Ron Van Clief I learned his Chinese Goju System. Although I did have some prior experience in Wing Chun Kung Fu and Jiu Jitsu, it was under his personal guidance that the essence of martial arts was unveiled to me. From these insights I was inspired to reach advanced levels of training.

A violent environment had been a normal part of my youth, and as a result of many physical altercations I became a fairly competent street fighter; my interest in martial arts grew mainly from curiosity about their history and character-building aspect, rather than from an urgent need to learn self-defense techniques. The more I advanced in rank and deepened my understanding of the history and philosophy of martial arts, the more I realized that there were important elements missing in our contemporary approach to training.

What I discovered is that traditionally martial arts training had placed equal emphasis on developing combat skills and nurturing the spirit of the aspiring student. Unfortunately the study of the healing arts, the practice of meditation, and the use of herbs—which were all important parts of development—are noticeably absent from modern martial arts training. On many occasions Shidoshi Van Clief and I discussed the views of ancient martial artists, who in their wisdom had recognized the importance of combining all these elements. The ancients realized that beyond the obvious benefits of herbs to health, energy levels, and injury management, integrating the study of healing arts with the practice of meditation offered other, more subtle benefits such as the increased sensitivity to pain and suffering that seems to be inherent in healers and the healing arts, and a raising of consciousness that can contribute to heightened spiritual development.

What appears to happen as a result of integrating these ancient arts can best be described as a refining of temperament and a harnessing of the aggressive tendencies that are sometimes accentuated through martial arts practice. Perhaps the powerful way that this integrated study can mitigate an individual's violent or aggressive tendencies occurs because, philosophically, such study is a manifestation of the yin-yang theory of opposites in balance—in which the yin (soft or healing arts) blends with the yang (hard or martial arts).

On a spiritual level, twenty years of studying these two ancient arts, combined with daily meditation, has convinced me that such study does indeed harmonize the emotions and provide a kind of reverence for life that is essential to anyone learning the skills of unarmed combat, which ultimately confers the ability to seriously injure or kill another human being. On a practical level, I attribute my overall good health and lack of any permanent injuries to the effectiveness of Chinese herbs, which I have used throughout my many years of training.

Therefore, I encourage all martial artists who are interested in experiencing firsthand the wisdom embodied in the traditional approach to martial arts training to consider making the study of healing arts, the practice of meditation, and the use of herbs parts of their martial arts practice.

I'd like to conclude with an excerpt from "Chinese Goju Virtues." Conceived by Shidoshi Ron Van Clief, Grandmaster of the Chinese Goju System, "Chinese Goju Virtues" serve as a guide or frame of reference to govern the moral character of everyone who studies the Chinese Goju style. I have always been inspired by them and have attempted to apply these principles whenever it has been necessary to use my martial skills.

Chinese Goju is my secret
I bear no arms
May God help me
If I ever have to use my art . . .

Yodan Thomas Richard Joiner
Fourth-Degree Black Belt
Oakland, California

A Brief Discussion
of the
Historical
Relationship
between
the Healing and
the Martial Arts

Because of the violence normally associated with the martial arts it would not be unreasonable to assume that early martial artists were members of either the palace guard, imperial troops, or some other quasi-military organization. Curiously, however, this is not the case.

More often they were physicians, Buddhist monks, herbalists, or Taoist priests whose martial arts training was centered on therapeutic movement and Chi Kung; the development of combat skills was a secondary consideration. And it is healing exercises such as Chi Kung—originally designed for maintaining health, calming the mind, and increasing longevity—that were the basis for the modern martial arts.

Over the past five thousand years, however, the character of martial arts has undergone a complete and somewhat troubling transformation. Original health concerns have given way to a total preoccupation with learning techniques whose only purpose is to injure, maim, or kill. Throughout their early history the Chinese martial arts' relationships with traditional Chinese medicine, herbology, religion, and philosophy were well established. These relationships, which were once integral to the practice of martial arts, have been steadily compromised in the name of progress.

Like all aspects of Chinese culture, the martial arts were once governed by the cosmological influences that emphasize harmony and balance in all issues pertaining to life. Ever conscious of the need to maintain equilibrium by mitigating the violent nature of martial arts, it was not uncommon at advanced levels of training for the *sifu* (teacher) to talk more about history, philosophy, and ethical and spiritual values than "kicking ass."

Although the credit for founding Chinese martial arts has been properly attributed to the Chan Buddhist monk Bodhidharma, it is in fact the Taoists who have been the chief promoters of strict adherence to the principles of harmony, which are represented in yin-yang theory, by incorporating the use of herbs and the practice of therapeutic exercise with the practice of martial arts. This integration of cosmic forces is critical. While there is no denying that combat is violent, combining it with healing practice serves to minimize its savagery.

In addition to creating what some consider the premier martial art "The Grand Ultimate Fist" (better known as Tai Chi Chuan), Taoists' use of movement to cure illness has always coincided with their use of botanicals (plants and herbs) to enhance training and treating disease. Tai Chi is undoubtedly one of Taoism's most important contributions to the Chinese martial arts. Equal in terms of its health benefits and the effectiveness of its martial applications, Tai Chi Chuan personifies the concept of balance by combining both healing and martial elements within the same style. For this reason Tai Chi is considered a "complete" system.

Whether it should be considered superior to all other martial arts styles is debatable. Serious martial arts study soon reveals that there is no "best" system; all styles have something to offer. All, however, are not as balanced as Tai Chi. Healing is an issue whose importance is often overlooked, especially by practitioners of external martial arts.

The preoccupation of these external arts with physical strength and the development of external physical structures, which is evidenced by the muscularity and callused hands of their practitioners, contrasts strikingly with internal styles that emphasize developing chi (vital energy) along with honing psychic or mental sensitivities. Traditionally it was believed that these more subtle qualities were developed through meditation, therapeutic exercise, and sexual alchemical processes. It was also believed that this development could be assisted by taking certain pharmaceutical concoctions (herbs). Although internal development is said to be somewhat slower than external, the effectiveness of an art developed in such a manner is unquestionable, as is the possibility of being able to practice it well into advanced age. In fact, health and longevity—issues given little consideration by modernists—were the predominant issues among ancient martial artists.

In the centuries that have transpired since the martial arts' beginnings there have been many changes. Conspicuously absent today are the early secret societies, strict adherence to philosophical guidelines, and fundamental relationship with healing arts. Regrettably, these all have given way to Kung Fu's enormous popularity and worldwide commercial acceptance.

The gradual erosion of principles and disintegration of traditional relationships that occurred over several centuries have become increasingly noticeable in the last fifty years. And although the decline has occurred to a greater extent in the West it has also become apparent in China, diminishing the value of what was once considered a national treasure. Modern martial artists have become mere shadows of their ancient predecessors.

Fortunately, there are also some encouraging signs. There is increasing evidence that public interest in therapeutic exercise in general and Chi Kung in particular is on the rise. In the United States traditional Chinese medicine is the most widely used alternative form of medical treatment—second only to traditional Western medicine. Also, more than twenty-five years after the death of Bruce Lee some believe that a martial arts renaissance is on the horizon. Finally, and perhaps most important, although few in number there is a select group of martial arts masters who continue to practice on a high level. These rare individuals, who usually prefer to operate under a cloak of anonymity, are the keepers of the flame, avoiding the fanfare and notoriety frequently bestowed on those who are less deserving and in no way representative of true martial artists.

For those of us who love martial arts and have adopted them as a way of life, the journey that is required to achieve excellence is indeed long and arduous. This is why it is important occasionally to pause and look back—to briefly reexamine the lives of some warriors, priests, monks, and healers. Reconsidering the principles and standards that they established many centuries ago is a source of inspiration.

Bodhidharma (P'u Ti Ta Mo) (448-527 C.E.)

Despite the uncertainty surrounding the beginning of the Chinese martial arts, it is generally accepted by most modern scholars that the principles of modern martial arts were advanced by the twenty-eighth patriarch, Chan Buddhist monk Bodhidharma, during the sixth century. History tells us that at the Shaolin Monastery, where monks toiled as scribes translating hundred of sacred scriptures into Chinese, this spiritual eccentric introduced the therapeutic exercises for strengthening the body and mind that are at the root of Chinese martial arts. In addition to these early calisthenics, Bodhidharma introduced self-defense movements from his vast knowledge of Indian fighting systems. This marked the beginning of Shaolin Temple Boxing.

Two of the most important forms that were practiced are the now-famous Muscle/Tendon Change and Marrow Washing (Chi Kung), and the Eighteen Lo Han Shou, better known as the Eighteen Buddha Hand. Strictly speaking, the exercises were not specifically designed for boxing; their primary purpose was the cultivation of chi, which could be used to advance longevity, maintain health, and contribute to spiritual development.

Although it is generally agreed that some forms of boxing did exist prior to the arrival of Bodhidharma, documentary evidence to support these claims is unavailable. It is known, however, that the essence of the great master's art was absorbed, enriched, and refined by succeeding Chan masters until it became the powerful Shaolin Temple Boxing that is commonly referred to as Shaolin Chuan (Shaolin Fist) or Shaolin Ch'uan Fa—(The Way of the Shaolin Fist). Some consider this the first documented martial arts system.

Emperor Shen Nong (2737-2697 B.C.E)

This divine architect of Chinese herbology is credited with, among other things, inventing the wooden plow and teaching the Chinese people the art of agriculture. Both inventions improved the quality of life; before Shen Nong's reign there was only hunting, fishing, raising animals, and foraging. Perfecting the art of agriculture provided more leisure time, which in turn allowed more time for social and cultural activities.

Shen Nong's most notable contribution, however, was founding (through experimentation and the tasting of hundreds of botanical substances) the traditional Chinese herbal system.

He is also credited with introducing tea drinking to Chinese culture. This was an important discovery when you consider that along with medicinal wine, tea is one of the earliest forms of herbal preparation. It is unquestionably the most popular.

The results of Shen Nong's herbal experiments were recorded in the *Shen Nong Ben Cao Jing* (Shen Nong Herbal Classic). Published around 200 B.C., *Shen Nong Ben Cao Jing* is considered the earliest classic on the subject of Chinese herbal medicine. Although there is no historical evidence of Shen Nong's direct involvement in the martial arts, he discovered the herbs that have been used for nearly five millennia to promote longevity, enhance training, maintain health, and treat martial arts injuries.

Hua To (136-220 C.E.)

Without a doubt one of the most celebrated physicians in Chinese history, Hua To was a skilled acupuncturist and Chinese herbalist who is also credited with introducing the concept and use of oral anesthesia while performing surgical procedures.

His advanced ideas concerning the relationships among exercise, nutrition, and preventative medicine were best represented through a series of exercises that he called "Five Animals Play." Hua To maintained that these simple exercises would evoke perspiration, which would cleanse the body and stimulate the appetite, resulting in the consumption of invigorating and health-promoting nourishment. These therapeutic movements were created from his observations of five animals: the tiger, deer, bear, ape, and bird. Although these exercises were not designed to enhance martial skills, they can be considered the initiators of later forms of Kung Fu based on animal movements.

According to legend Hua To was summoned by the imperial throne to treat the prime minister's unrelenting headaches. Hua To suggested cutting a hole in his skull to release the toxic fluids that he believed to be the cause. Thinking that it was a plot to murder him, the prime minister ordered that Hua To be imprisoned and subsequently sentenced him to death. Realizing that his execution was imminent, Hua To committed suicide by drinking poison.

Emperor Huang Ti (2696-2598 B.C.E.)

Huang Ti, perhaps better known as the Yellow Emperor, was the revolutionary leader credited with unifying the warring states into what is now known as China. He was also an accomplished classical Chinese wrestler, and there are reports of a power struggle in which he used his considerable martial skills to defeat his archenemy, Chi Yu.

Although his contributions toward advancing Chinese history and culture are numerous, Huang Ti is frowned upon by many historians because of his heavy-handed use of imperial power. Notable among these repressive acts were orders to burn all books in an attempt to control the minds of his subjects, and the building of the Great Wall of China using forced labor.

Despite these controversies, though, the Yellow Emperor's place in the annals of Chinese history is firmly established, mainly because of his authorship of *Nei Ching Su Wan* (The Yellow Emperor's Classic of Internal Medicine), said to be the oldest existing Chinese medical text.

It is also noted in historical accounts that Huang Ti was obsessed with finding a means to achieve immortality. He used pharmaceutical concoctions (herbal formulas) that were developed as a result of Taoist experiments, as well as practicing therapeutic exercises, in his efforts toward that end. No such elixir was developed, and the emperor died during his search.

Most great thinkers concur about the importance of combining the old with the new, history with the present, and the past with the future. The legendary figures whose lives I have briefly discussed all made immeasurable contributions to the development of both healing and martial arts; without them the martial arts we know would not exist. Their influence can be seen in every form of these arts. I feel that these figures, as well as many others I have not mentioned, should be honored.

Methods of Herb Preparation

Herbs can be prepared and used in a variety of ways. Understandably, when we choose a method of preparation convenience is usually our main concern. Prepackaged herbal formulas in pill form, or patent formulas, are readily available in most Chinatowns or from Chinese herbal mail-order houses. Patent medicines, the most convenient form, include instructions for use as well as recommended dosage.

Still, my personal experience has been that each method of preparation has a specific application for which it is best suited, and that using raw herbs prepared by the methods I will discuss in the following pages is more effective than using patent formulas. Raw herbs have greater potency—plus in the long term they can be less expensive. Admittedly, some methods of preparation require more effort than others, but their aesthetic and therapeutic benefits greatly outweigh any inconvenience.

For each raw herb formula I discuss in this book I recommend one of three methods of preparation: decoction, medicinal wine, or pills and capsules. Following are detailed instructions on how to prepare each.

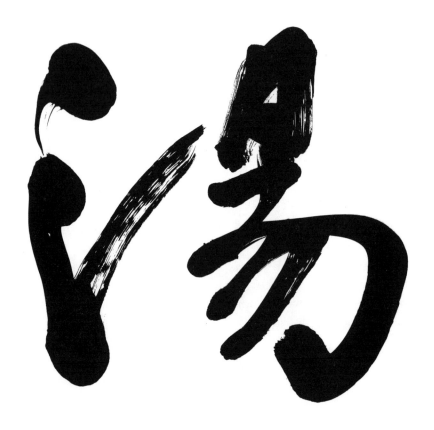

TANG
DECOCTION

Decoction

Tea drinking is such an important part of Asian culture that it is not surprising that preparing a decoction (basically a tea) is the most popular way to use Chinese herbs.

Decoctions are especially effective for acute disorders because they are quickly assimilated into the bloodstream, so their healing effects are felt more rapidly. You must use the decoction method for formulas that include harder plant materials (such as roots or bark) that must be cooked to extract their therapeutic properties.

Although preparation is quite simple, there are several important points to remember:

- Never cook in an aluminum pot. Use porcelain, Pyrex, enamel, or glass. These substances are preferable to any metal, including stainless steel.
- When preparing a decoction, first bring the water to a rolling boil and then add the herbs; this is necessary in order to extract their therapeutic properties.
- Always simmer the decoction over a low flame.
- Never store the decoction in a plastic container.

How to Prepare a Decoction

1. Bring the specified quantity of room-temperature water to a boil in a large pot.
2. Add the herbs, stir, and return to a boil; lower the heat to simmer and cover the pot.
3. Simmer over a low flame for 30 minutes.
4. Remove the pot from the heat with the lid on. Allow the cooked tea to cool in the pot for another 30 minutes.
5. Strain off the herbs and discard them.
6. Place the strained herbal tea in a glass container for storage.

To make enough decoction to last for one day, add 1 to 2 ounces of fresh herbs to 24 ounces of boiling water. Continue as instructed above. After the cooking process, the water will be reduced to approximately 16 ounces. Drink $1/2$ cup (or 4 ounces) at room

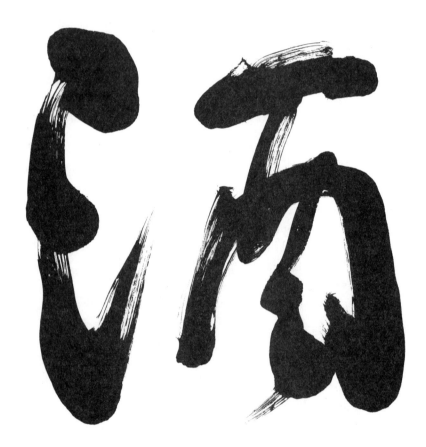

JIU
WINE

temperature 3 times daily (in the morning, afternoon, and evening).

If you want to make up larger quantities of an herbal formula—enough to last for several days or a week—simply double, triple, or quadruple the water-to-herb ratio and prepare as described above. Drink the decocted tea at room temperature, but refrigerate all leftovers. Herbal decoctions can be stored in the refrigerator for 10 to 14 days.

Taoists believe that neither hot nor cold is desirable for ingestion; a tepid or neutral temperature is recommended. After preparing an herbal decoction, then, let it come to room temperature before drinking it.

Medicinal Wine

The ancient practice of aging herbs in alcohol is by far the simplest and, by some accounts, the oldest known method for making medicinal preparations. Make a *jui dan* (medicinal wine) by leaving herbs in an alcohol solution until the herbal properties are extracted or drawn out by the alcohol. The spirit or wine itself is considered to possess nourishing, blood-invigorating properties that enhance the therapeutic effects of the herbs prepared with it.

When jui dan preparations are intended for internal consumption, sweet rice wine or vodka are the spirits of choice. If you use the latter, you can add honey to improve the taste. The alcohol should be no more than 80 proof. For preparations such as liniments that are applied externally, on the other hand, use brandy, ethanol, or rectified turpentine. Add the herbs to a fifth (liter) of alcohol or spirit.

How to Prepare a Medicinal Wine
1. Uncap the bottle of alcohol and pour off enough to make room for the specified amount of herbs.
2. Add the herbs and recap the bottle.
3. Store it in a cool, dry place for a minimum of 60 to 90 days.
4. Gently shake the bottle once a week during this time.

When the aging process has been completed, do not discard the

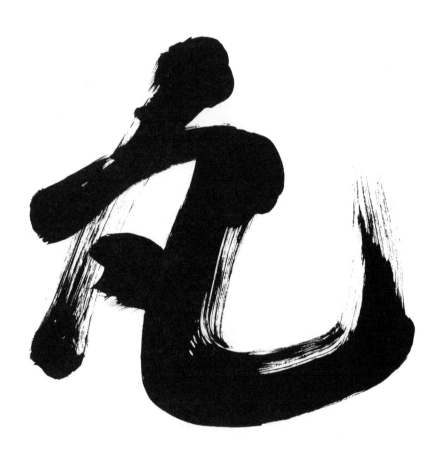

WAN

PILLS

herbs—they should remain in the bottle until all of the wine has been consumed. The longer the medicinal wine is stored (or aged), the more potent it will become. It is not uncommon to age a medicinal wine for as long as one year.

The standard quantity of herbs to use to prepare a medicinal wine is $1^1/_2$ to $2^1/_2$ ounces of fresh herbs to 1 fifth or liter of spirit. Once the jui dan has aged properly, the standard dose to drink is 1 ounce of wine at room temperature 3 times daily (in the morning, afternoon, and evening). You can dilute the medicinal wine in 4 ounces of tepid water or drink it straight up.

Instructions for the application of liniments prepared by this method are given with each specific liniment formula.

Pills and Capsules

To make pills or capsules from a single herb or from a multiple-herb formula, the herb(s) must first be ground down into a fine powder. You can do this in a household blender or by purchasing the herbs powdered from the herb store. For a small fee, herb stores will grind the herbs for you.

Many herbal formulas that are made into pills and capsules require you to dip an herb first in vinegar or another substance. To do this, simply dip the herb into cider or distilled vinegar as many times as instructed.

Traditionally, most herbal formulas were prepared as pills; if you prefer, however, you may prepare the herbs in capsule form without compromising their effectiveness.

How to Prepare Pills
1. Mix the herbal ingredients together and grind them into a fine powder.
2. Combine the powder with a viscous or sticky medium (honey is preferred).
3. Take a small amount of the mixture into the palm of your hand and roll it into the shape of a bean or pea.

4. Set the pill on a flat surface to dry.

5. When dry, store the pills in a glass jar and refrigerate.

How to Prepare Capsules

1. Purchase empty gelatin capsules from a health food store (the preferred size is 00).

2. Grind the herbal formula into a fine powder and put it into the capsules.

3. The caps can be stored indefinitely in a tightly sealed container.

Instructions on dosage are given with the description of specific formulas.

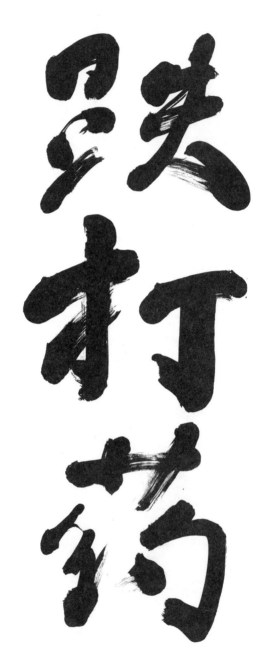

跌打药

TIEH TA
HIT MEDICINE

2
Injury-
Management
Formulas

It is regrettable that most martial artists today lack the ability to administer what is considered basic first aid while practicing a sport that by its very nature makes its participants more susceptible to trauma (which is most often minor, but occasionally produces what are considered major injuries). Traditionally, however, martial artists were well versed in treating and managing many of the injuries that were sustained in training or combat. A working knowledge of botanicals that could be found in the field (wild in nature) and used for treating a variety of wounds and injuries was an integral part of field training. These materials were often self-administered, but at other times used to treat injured comrades. The ability to identify and successfully use plant medicines was in many cases a matter of life and death.

This ancient tradition, although no longer entirely practical (in terms of saving lives), is nonetheless a part of martial arts that should be preserved. It still has both aesthetic and practical benefits—which are in jeopardy of being lost because so few modern martial artists are familiar with the large variety of herbs available or how they can be used to treat the wide range of injuries that can occur during sparring, or simply as a result of the rigors of daily training.

While it is a fairly common practice to use the herbal liniments known as *dit da jow* to prevent injuries while conditioning the hands and other parts of the body used for striking (head, elbows, forearms, shin), the modern martial artist is usually uninformed about the traditional use of herbs for managing martial arts injuries. Most have a limited knowledge of herbs and are only familiar with the more popular ones, such as ginseng.

As you can imagine, the simulated fighting or sparring *(kimute)* that is necessary to develop and perfect technique also increases the possibility of minor injuries as well as some of a more serious nature. In this chapter I present herbal formulas for treating both major and minor injuries common to practice (broken bones, cuts, abrasions, internal and external hemorrhage, contusions, muscle strain, tendon pulls, and so on). There are even formulas for restoring consciousness after a knockout!

Herbs That Stop Bleeding

All combat sports—martial arts, boxing, and the like—are commonly referred to as blood sports because of the trauma and bleeding that are inherent to them. Bleeding, which can be external (outside of the body), or internal (inside the body), is a result of blunt trauma caused by strikes or kicks from fists, feet, elbows, knees, shins, or head butts. Certain areas of the body are more likely to bleed, either internally or externally. For instance, strikes to bony areas such as the face normally produce external bleeding (common examples are nosebleeds or cuts above the eyes), while strikes to the body or torso are more likely to cause internal bleeding (common examples are spleen ruptures or kidney abrasions).

The herbal formulas used to treat such injuries are known as blood formulas and are used for all kinds of traumatic bleeding, including simple nosebleeds, cuts, coughing or vomiting up blood, and blood in the urine. These formulas stop bleeding, speed up coagulation of the blood, eliminate blood clots, and restore normal blood flow. They can be simple single-herb formulas or more complex ones that involve as many as a dozen herbs. As you might imagine, there is a correlation between the severity of an injury and the complexity of the formula used for treating it. Generally speaking, simple injuries (superficial cuts, nosebleeds) can be treated with less complicated formulas, while severe injuries (like broken bones) will usually require a formula with a greater number of ingredients.

Blood Formulas

Raw Form Preparations

Tian Chi Ginseng (pseudo ginseng)
Zi Su Ye (perilla leaf)
Shaolin Wan Nang Zhi Xue San (Ten Thousand Abilities to Stop Bleeding Powder)
Shi Zhu Xue Tang (Treatment for Unstoppable Bleeding Formula)
Shih Chuan Xiu Xue Tang (General-Purpose Stop Bleeding Formula)

Patent Formulas

Yunnan Bai Yao (Yunnan White Medicine)

TIAN CHI GINSENG

PSEUDO GINSENG

An example of a single-herb formula that is useful whenever there is bleeding—internal or external—is Tian Chi Ginseng (also known as pseudo ginseng). The raw powdered herb can be applied directly to an open wound or abrasion to arrest external bleeding. To stop internal bleeding mix 1.5 grams of raw herb powder with approximately 4 ounces of room-temperature sweet rice wine and drink.

Analysis of the Herbs in This Formula

The herb Tian Chi Ginseng stops bleeding and transforms con-gealed blood. It is used for internal and external bleeding, includ-ing vomiting blood, nosebleed, and blood in the urine or stool. Because this herb can stop bleeding without causing congealed blood, it is very widely used. It is the herb of choice for traumatic injuries and can be used internally as well as externally (topically).

Caution

It is important to note that Tian Chi Ginseng should never be taken internally by a pregnant woman. It could harm the fetus.

Zi Su Ye

PERILLA LEAF

Another example of the single-herb approach to first aid is the use of the herb Zi Su Ye to stop bleeding from the nose. This large, leafy herb is used as follows: Instruct the patient to tilt his or her head back and to breathe through the mouth, then tear off a large portion of the leaf and insert the Zi Su Ye into the nostril, filling the nasal passage entirely, and apply direct pressure (pinch the nose) for 5 to 10 minutes.

If there is still bleeding after the first application, repeat the procedure. If bleeding persists beyond 20 to 30 minutes seek professional help.

Analysis of the Herbs in This Formula

The herb Zi Su Ye is mainly used to correct digestive disturbances, as well as being effective in stopping nosebleeds.

Shaolin Wan Nang Zhi Xue San

TEN THOUSAND ABILITIES TO STOP BLEEDING POWDER

As I mentioned earlier, injuries of a more serious nature generally require more complex formulas. An example would be cases involving both internal and external bleeding with accompanying pain and bruising. For generations martial artists have used a formula called Shaolin Wan Nang Zhi Xue San (Ten Thousand Abilities to Stop Bleeding Powder) to treat serious traumatic injuries. While this formula is similar to Tian Chi Ginseng in that it can be used both internally and externally, its added ingredients make it applicable to a broader range of symptoms, including pain, infection, bruising, and of course internal and external bleeding.

Herbal Ingredients

GRAMS NEEDED	CHINESE NAME	ENGLISH TRANSLATION
30	Ma Bo	puffball fruit
30	Sheng Di Huang	Chinese foxglove root
30	Bai Ji	bletilla rhizome
30	Jin Yin Hua	honeysuckle flower
15	Xue Yu Tan	charred human hair
9	Da Huang	rhubarb root
9	Zhi Zi	gardenia fruit
9	Huang Bai	cork tree bark
9	Huang Lian	golden thread
15	Er Cha	cutch paste
12	Ru Xiang (dip in vinegar 1 time)	frankincense
12	Mo Yao	myrrh
10	Xue Jie	dragon's blood resin
15	Zi Ran Ton (dip in vinegar 7 times)	pyrite
3	She Xiang	deer gland secretions
3	Bing Pian	camphor resin

Analysis of the Herbs in This Formula

Zhi Zi and Sheng Di Huang cool the blood. Jin Yin Hua, Huang Lian, Er Cha, and Huang Bai clear infection; the ability to arrest bleeding is a somewhat minor function. Bai Ji is used for bleeding from the lungs (coughing up blood) and stomach (vomiting blood). Of the remaining herbs in this formula (Da Huang, Xue Yu Tan, and Ma Bo) are primarily used to stop bleeding, including intestinal bleeding and blood in the urine, while Xue Jie, Zi Ran Ton, Ru Xiang, She Xiang, and Bing Pian alleviate pain, dissolve clots, reduce swelling, and promote healing.

Recommended Method of Preparation

To properly prepare this formula, you must first grind the herbs into a fine powder. Pour this onto an open, bleeding wound to stop external bleeding, or mix 1.5 grams of it with 4 ounces of room-temperature sweet rice wine and drink to stop internal bleeding.

Recommended Dosage

Use 1.5 grams of the powdered herb a day for 1 to 2 days for both internal and external application.

Caution

If bleeding persists, seek the advice of a physician!

Shi Zhu Xue Tang

TREATMENT FOR UNSTOPPABLE BLEEDING FORMULA

It has been my experience that certain techniques are more likely to cause trauma that results in bleeding. One is the technique called "iron elbow" or "monkey elbow," which has been associated with broken ribs, kidney lacerations, and spleen ruptures. Shi Zhu Xue Tang is useful for treating internal hemorrhage anywhere in the body that has been caused by punches, kicks, or elbow strikes, as well as strikes from blunt objects.

Herbal Ingredients

GRAMS NEEDED	CHINESE NAME	ENGLISH TRANSLATION
18	Dang Gui	tang-kuei root
9	Bai Shao	white peony root
12	E Jiao	donkey skin glue
9	Bai Ji	bletilla rhizome
3	Hong Hua	safflower
6	Jie Geng	balloonflower root
6	Zhi Qiao	bitter orange fruit
3	Tian Chi Ginseng	pseudo ginseng root
30	Sheng Di Huang	Chinese foxglove root
12	Hei Jing Jie	blackened jingjie
9	Bai Shuang	fumaria dust
30	brown sugar	raw brown sugar

Analysis of the Herbs in This Formula

When combined, the herbs Tian Chi Ginseng, Bai Ji, E Jiao, and Bai Shuang will powerfully arrest internal bleeding. Dang Gui and Bai Shao both enrich the blood and stop pain, while Hong Hua circulates the blood and resolves blood clots.

Sheng Di Huang cools the blood, Jie Geng discharges pus and abscesses, and Hei Jing Jie and Zhi Qiao are auxiliary herbs that assist in arresting bleeding. Brown sugar is used to harmonize (improve the taste of) the other herbs in the formula.

Recommended Method of Preparation
Prepare a decoction. (See chapter 1 for instructions.)

Recommended Dosage:
Drink 4 ounces of tea (prepared herbal decoction) 3 times daily for 1 to 2 days.

Caution
It is important to note the Tian Chi Ginseng should never be taken internally by a pregnant woman. It could harm the fetus.

If bleeding persists, seek the advice of a physician!

Shih Chuan Xiu Xue Tang
GENERAL-PURPOSE STOP BLEEDING FORMULA

An excellent herbal formula to use whenever someone is "all beaten up" is Shih Chuan Xiu Xue Tang. This can be used when there is localized bleeding, bruising, and swelling. "Localized bleeding" refers to minor injuries such as those that might be suffered during full-contact sparring: bloody nose, black eyes, scrapes, bruises, abrasions, and lacerations.

Note that the use of Shih Chuan Xiu Xue Tang satisfies an interesting Chinese medical principle of first aid that states that by taking internal medicine you expedite external healing.

Herbal Ingredients

GRAMS NEEDED	CHINESE NAME	ENGLISH TRANSLATION
15	Dang Gui	tang-kuei root
9	Chuan Xiong	lovage root
9	Hong Hua	safflower
6	Chen Pi	tangerine peel
4.5	Mu Xiang	costus root
6	Zhi Qiao	bitter orange fruit
9	Tao Ren	peach kernel
6	Mu Tong	wood with holes
6	Ru Xiang (dip in vinegar 1 time)	frankincense
4.5	Mo Yao	myrrh
6	Gan Cao	licorice root

Analysis of the Herbs in This Formula

Dang Gui stops pain and enriches the blood, while Hong Hua and Chuan Xiong circulate it. Tao Ren circulates the blood as well as assisting Mo Yao in eliminating blood clots. Chen Pi and Mu Xiang circulate the chi, and Mu Tong unblocks blood vessels. Zhi Qiao is an auxiliary herb that stops bleeding, and Ru Xiang reduces swelling, promotes healing, and alleviates pain. Gan Cao is used to harmonize (improve the taste of) the other herbs in this formula.

Recommended Method of Preparation
Make a decoction. (See chapter 1 for instructions.)

Recommended Dosage
Drink 4 ounces of herbal tea (decoction) 3 times daily for 1 to 2 days.

Caution
If bleeding persists, seek the advice of a physician!

YUNNAN BAI YAO PATENT FORMULA

YUNNAN WHITE MEDICINE
ALSO KNOWN AS YUN NAN PAIYAO

Among the prepared herbal formulas (or patent formulas) that stop bleeding, Yunnan Bai Yao is perhaps the most famous. One of its main ingredients is Tian Chi Ginseng.

This formula is well known for its ability to stop bleeding from incisions, stab wounds, knife cuts, gunshot wounds, bruises, contusions, and so on. Yunnan Bai Yao should be included in the first-aid kit of every dojo.

To stop bleeding with this formula, first take the small red pill that comes in every package and then pour the loose powder directly onto the wound. Be sure to use enough powder to cover the wound completely.

Caution

It is important to note that Yunnan Bai Yao and Tian Chi Ginseng should never be taken internally by a pregnant woman. They could harm the fetus.

The herbs and patent medicines mentioned in the last few pages have been used in traditional Chinese medicine and martial arts for centuries to arrest bleeding. Although there are several other formulas in Chinese herbology that fall within this category of herbs that stop bleeding, I have not included them here because for the most part they are simply variations of the previously mentioned formulas, with Tian Chi Ginseng as their main ingredient. Traditionally, herbs that stop bleeding were especially useful in martial arts schools known for heavy sparring (because of the likelihood of cuts and abrasions), and in schools or styles where the use of bladed weapons was taught.

Herbs That Heal Broken and Fractured Bones

Although they can hardly be considered a common occurrence, serious injuries do occasionally happen during martial arts training. Among the more serious are broken bones. The body is made up of a disproportionate number of small bones compared with the number of large ones. Ironically the weapons most used by the martial artist, the hands, contain many of these small bones, increasing their likelihood of being injured. By far more fractured bones occur in the hands during sparring, actual combat, and conditioning than in any other body part.

The legs, which contain the largest bones in the body, are a common point of attack by sweeps and kicks. Although surprisingly resilient, they are after the hands the site where fractures most frequently occur.

Broken bones are perhaps the most debilitating injury that a martial artist can suffer. When such injuries occur during combat, the loss of a weapon can put the combatant at a serious disadvantage. This speaks strongly to the importance of developing a daily regime of conditioning both hands and shins.

After a broken bone has been set and a cast applied there are several herbal formulas that hasten recovery.

Herbal Formulas That Heal Fractured Bones

Raw Form Preparations

Gu Zhe Tang (Bone-Break Formula)
Cheung Gu Wan (Penetrating Bone Pills)
Jie Gu Tang (Connect the Bones Elixir)

Patent Formulas

Chin Koo Tieh Shang Wan (Muscle and Bone Traumatic Injury Pills)
Gu Zhe Cuo Shang San (Bones Broken Bruised Capsules)

Gu Zhe Tang

BONE-BREAK FORMULA

Gu Zhe Tang can be used for broken bones anywhere in the body. It is especially useful to martial artists who sustain broken bones in the hand as a result of iron-palm training or from practicing *shirwara,* more commonly known as breaking technique. Shirwara is practiced in some styles of Karate and featured prominently in the Korean art of Tae Kwon Do. It is practiced to toughen the striking surfaces of the body (such as the hands, feet, and head) and to demonstrate power, focus, and the correct application of force.

In order for broken bones to heal properly, circulation must be restored to the damaged area and maintained throughout the healing period. Gu Zhe Tang is well known for its ability to promote the circulation of chi and blood through the joints and bones.

Herbal Ingredients

GRAMS NEEDED	CHINESE NAME	ENGLISH TRANSLATION
3	Xu Duan	teasel root
1.5	Shu Di Huang	wine-cooked Chinese foxglove root
1.5	Dang Gui	tang-kuei root
1.5	Niu Xi	ox-knee root
1.5	Wu Jia Pi	five-bark root
1.5	Shan Zhu Yu	dried cornelian cherry
1.5	Du Zhong	eucommia bark
1.5	Bai Shao	white peony root
1.5	Fu Ling	tuckahoe root
1	Qing Pi	green tangerine peel

Analysis of the Herbs in This Formula

Xu Duan, the major (or emperor) herb in this formula, is known for connecting broken bones, promoting circulation, and strengthening the sinews. Its bone-connecting effects are supported by Niu

Xi, which, in addition to strengthening the bones and sinews, benefits the joints. Du Zhong and Wu Jia Pi also assist in strengthening the bones and sinews. Dang Gui, Bai Shao, and Shu Di Huang all enrich the blood and stop pain. Shan Zhu Yu, Fu Ling, and Qing Pi settle the stomach and mitigate the harshness of some of the other herbs in the formula.

Recommended Method of Preparation
Make a decoction. (See chapter 1 for instructions.)

Recommended Dosage
Drink 4 ounces of tea (decocted herbs) at room temperature 3 times daily until bones are healed.

Caution
This formula should be taken until recovery is complete. Do not use this formula if you are pregnant. It could harm the fetus.

CHEUNG GU WAN
PENETRATING BONE PILLS

The formula Cheung Gu Wan is said to date all the way back to the Han dynasty (25–220 C.E.). It was often used by ancient martial artists to treat broken bones. The herbs in this formula must be mixed together, then ground into a fine powder and made into pills—hence the name Penetrating Bone Pills.

In addition to its use for fractures this formula was famous among ancient martial artists for its bone-strengthening ability. Its herbs help to correct the flow of chi through fractured bones and to increase bone strength and density.

Herbal Ingredients

GRAMS NEEDED	CHINESE NAME	ENGLISH TRANSLATION
3	Sheng Di Huang	Chinese foxglove root
3	Bai Shao	white peony root
1.5	Mu Dan Pi	peony root bark
1.5	Hong Hua	safflower
1.5	Da Huang	rhubarb root
1.5	Gou Gu	dog bone

Analysis of the Herbs in This Formula
Sheng Di Huang and Mu Dan Pi both cool the blood. Hong Hua circulates the blood and is assisted by Da Huang in eliminating blood clots. Bai Shao enriches the blood, and Gou Gu strengthens the bones and sinews.

Recommended Method of Preparation
Mix the herbs, grind into a fine powder, and make into pills. (See chapter 1 for complete instructions on how to prepare herbal formulas as pills.)

Traditionally, this formula was prepared as in pill form, but if you prefer you may put the ground herbs into capsules.

Recommended Dosage

Take 3 pills or capsules 3 times daily, 30 minutes after meals (breakfast, lunch, and dinner). Swallow with tepid water, as if you are taking an aspirin.

Caution

The instructions for using Cheung Gu Wan specifically state that self-treatment should not exceed 10 consecutive days!

JIE GU TANG

CONNECT THE BONES ELIXIR

I consider myself extremely fortunate in that I have never person-ally suffered a fracture during my martial arts training. I have, however, witnessed several incidents of ribs being fractured in the dojo during full-contact sparring.

In addition to complaints about pain and discomfort, a com-mon complaint of everyone I have known who has suffered a bone break is the length of time required for healing. Jie Gu Tang is renowned for its ability to assist in this healing.

Herbal Ingredients

GRAMS NEEDED	CHINESE NAME	ENGLISH TRANSLATION
9	Dang Gui	tang-kuei root
9	Hong Hua	safflower
9	Tao Ren	peach kernel
9	Da Huang	rhubarb root
30	Ye Ju Hua	chrysanthemum flower
12	Mu Dan Pi	peony root bark
9	Yang Ti	goat hooves
6	Tu Bie Chong (remove head and legs)	wingless cockroach
4.5	Zi Ran Ton (dipped in vinegar 7 times)	pyrite
6	Gan Cao	licorice root

Analysis of the Herbs in This Formula

Dang Gui enriches the blood and alleviates pain, Da Huang assists Hong Hua and Tao Ren in circulating the blood and preventing clotting, Mu Dan Pi cools the blood, Ye Ju Hua prevents subepider-mal sores and infection. Yang Ti, Tu Bie Chong, and Zi Ran Ton all resolve clotting and are useful for contusions and fractures while promoting the healing of bones and sinews. Gan Cao harmonizes (improves the taste of) the other herbs in this formula.

Recommended Method of Preparation
Make a decoction. (See chapter 1 for instructions.)

Recommended Dosage
Drink 1 cup of tepid tea (from herbal decoction) once a day until the bones are healed.

———————

There are also several formulas available for those who prefer the convenience of buying prepackaged formulas in pill form. I'll describe the two that I consider best for healing fractured bones.

Chin Koo Tieh Shang Wan Patent Formula

MUSCLE AND BONE TRAUMATIC INJURY PILLS

ALSO KNOWN AS JIN GU DIE SHANG WAN

This is an excellent formula for speeding recovery from fractures. It will reduce pain and swelling and invigorate the blood and fluids while it strengthens the tendons and bones. Formulas like Chin Koo Tieh Shang Wan were traditionally used not only for treating injuries but also as training supplements (much the way that vitamins and minerals are used today) because of their ability to strengthen the tendons and bones.

This patent medicine comes in bottles of 120 small black pills, complete with instructions for dosage.

Caution

This formula should never be taken internally by a pregnant woman. It could harm the fetus.

Gu Zhe Cuo Shang San Patent formula

BONES BROKEN BRUISED CAPSULES
ALSO KNOWN AS FRACTURA PULVIS PILLS

Another formula that will help heal broken bones is Gu Zhe Cuo Shang San. It also has the ability to strengthen weak bones, stop pain, and reduce inflammation. This patent medicine comes in bottles of capsules with complete instructions on dosage.

Caution
This formula should never be taken internally by a pregnant woman. It could harm the fetus.

Herbs that Heal Strained and Torn Ligaments

Over the years I have known many misguided martial artists who, as a result of their preoccupation with muscle development, paid little attention to strengthening and developing the supporting structures—ligaments and tendons. The frequency of this oversight is substantiated by the high number of injuries involving sprained, strained, pulled, twisted, and torn ligaments and tendons. These fairly common injuries usually occur during training.

Ligaments—the fibrous tissues that connect bones to bones, undergo two common injuries: minor sprains and tears. Minor sprains are treated with ice to reduce swelling, then bandaged for support, followed by physical therapy when needed. The more serious torn ligament usually requires surgical repair, after which it is immobilized in a soft cast (to allow proper healing). Like a broken bone, a torn ligament requires a lengthy healing time, usually six to eight weeks.

Tendons, on the other hand, are fibrous cords connecting muscle to bone. Common injuries include ruptures and inflammation—what is called tendonitis. Occasionally tendons are severed; surgery is required to reconnect their torn ends. In some cases it is necessary to graft tendon from elsewhere in the body or from a donor's tendon in order to reconnect them. Treatment for ruptures and tendonitis consists of resting the affected body part, applying ice packs, and using herbal therapy to reduce inflammation, alleviate swelling, and restore normal blood flow.

Increased amounts of stretching, practicing Tai Chi Chuan, and using herbal supplements are some of the techniques recommended to develop and strengthen ligaments and tendons in an attempt to avoid injury.

Herbal Formulas That Aid Recovery from Torn Ligaments or Tendons

Raw Form Preparation

Qi Li San (Seven Thousandths of a Tael Powder)
Pang Xie Lao Wo Nui Tang (Prescription for Treatment of Injury to Tendons)
Shaolin Shuang Jin Xue Gu Dan (Shaolin Strengthen the Sinews and Connect the Bones Elixir)
Shaolin Zhan Jin Dan (Extend the Sinews Elixir)

Patent Formula

Qi Li San (Seven Thousandths of a Tael Powder)

QI LI SAN
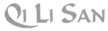

SEVEN THOUSANDTHS OF A TAEL POWDER

Martial artists know well that in order to excel they must spend an equal amount of time developing strength and flexibility. The body of the Karateka and Kung Fu practitioner *must* be flexible. Such suppleness can be acquired through a program of prescribed stretching exercises. Unfortunately, one of the features of rigorous flexibility training is the occasional sprained or torn ligament.

Qi Li San is renowned for its ability to reduce the healing time for a torn ligament. This formula will invigorate the blood, promote the movement of chi, and reduce swelling and pain.

Herbal Ingredients

GRAMS NEEDED	CHINESE NAME	ENGLISH TRANSLATION
30	Xue Jie	dragon's blood resin
4.5	Hong Hua	safflower
4.5	Ru Xiang	frankincense
4.5	Mo Yao	myrrh
.36	She Xiang	deer gland secretions
.36	Bing Pian	camphor resin
7.5	Er Cha	cutch paste
3.6	Zhu Sha	cinnabar

Analysis of the Herbs in This Formula

Hong Hua circulates the blood and prevents clotting. Ru Xiang, She Xiang, and Bing Pian all alleviate pain, dissolve blood clots, reduce swelling, and promote healing. Mo Yao also reduces swelling and alleviates pain. Er Cha primarily clears infection and has the minor ability to stop bleeding. Xue Jie can be used either internally or externally to stop bleeding; it will strengthen the sinews as well as being useful for treating symptoms related to injuries from falls, contusions, fractures, and sprains. Zhu Sha has a sedative effect.

Recommended Method of Preparation

Mix the herbs and then grind them into a fine powder.

Recommended Dosage

Mix 1.5 grams of powder with 4 ounces of sweet rice wine or warm water. Drink daily until healing is complete.

Qi Li San is also available in a prepared patent formula for those who prefer the convenience of using patent medicines. It is sold in powdered form in small glass vials; each vial contains 1.5 grams. Dosage instructions are included in the package.

Pang Xie Lao Wo Nui Tang

PRESCRIPTION FOR TREATMENT OF INJURY TO TENDONS

In this formula traditional Chinese medicine has an excellent remedy for the treatment of injured tendons and ligaments that, regrettably, many in Western culture find repulsive. I hope this aversion can be overcome, since the remedy is famed for its ability to provide quick relief.

A freshwater soft-shell crab, what the Chinese call *pang xie,* and a large snail known as *lao wo nui* are used. To prepare this formula, the snail is removed from its shell and then smashed. The crab, although left in its shell, is smashed as well. Then the two are mixed together and applied to the affected area. The area is covered with a broad, cloth bandage and then wrapped firmly with white gauze.

This formula will quickly reduce the swelling from strained tendons and ligaments. Discard it after the swelling is reduced.

SHAOLIN SHUANG JIN XUE GU DAN

SHAOLIN STRENGTHEN THE SINEWS AND CONNECT THE BONES ELIXIR

A useful formula for those who might be turned off by the preceding one is Shaolin Shuang Jin Xue Gu Dan. It strengthens the tendons and ligaments and shortens the healing time after an injury.

Herbal ingredients

GRAMS NEEDED	CHINESE NAME	ENGLISH TRANSLATION
60	Dang Gui	tang-kuei root
30	Chuan Xiong	lovage root
30	Bai Shao	white peony root
30	Shu Di Huang	wine-cooked Chinese foxglove root
30	Du Zhong	eucommia bark
60	Wu Jia Pi	five-bark root
90	Gu Sui Bu	mender of shattered bones rhizome
30	Gui Zhi	Saigon cinnamon twig
30	Tian Chi Ginseng	pseudo ginseng
30	Hu Gu	tiger bone*
60	Bu Gu Zhi	scuffy pea fruit
60	Tu Si Zi	dodder seeds
60	Dang Shen	relative root
30	Mu Gua	quince fruit
60	Liu Ji Nu	Liu's residing slave
90	Tu Bie Chong	wingless cockroach
30	Huang Qi	milk vetch root
60	Xu Duan	teasel root

* Tiger bone is an illegal substance in the United States. See pages 77–78 for more on this subject.

Analysis of the Herbs in This Formula

The herbs Dang Gui, Bai Shao, and Shu Di Huang all enrich the blood and stop pain, while Chuan Xiong, Gui Zhi, and Mu Gua circulate the blood. Du Zhong, Wu Jia Pi, and Hu Gu all strengthen bones and sinews. Xu Duan heals fractured bones. Tian Chi Ginseng and Bu Gu Zhi stop bleeding. Tu Si Zi assists in stopping bleeding, but its main function—along with Dang Shen and Huang Qi—is circulating the chi. Liu Ji Nu, Gu Sui Bu, and Tu Bie Chong all relieve pain, prevent blood clots, and accelerate healing.

Recommended Method of Preparation

Mix the herbs and grind them into a fine powder to be used as pills. (See chapter 1 for full instruction on how to prepare pills.) Traditionally, this formula was intended to be made into pills; if you prefer, however, you may prepare the herbs in capsule form.

Recommended Dosage

Take 1 pill twice a day, drunk with sweet rice wine at room temperature, until healing is complete.

Caution

Any formula containing Tian Chi Ginseng should not be used by a pregnant woman. It could harm the fetus!

SHAOLIN ZHAN JIN DAN

EXTEND THE SINEWS ELIXIR

This last formula used to treat ligaments and tendons is like a combination of all those previously mentioned. It was well known among ancient martial artists for its abilities to aid in the healing of strains and tears. Shaolin Zhan Jin Dan is considered especially useful for martial artists practicing styles that require a more rigorous stretching regimen, such as Wu Shu acrobatics, which requires astounding physical agility. Strains and tears of ligaments are likely to occur more frequently in these styles.

Herbal Ingredients

GRAMS NEEDED	CHINESE NAME	ENGLISH TRANSLATION
60	Dang Gui	tang-kuei root
60	Chuan Xiong	lovage root
45	Hong Hua	safflower
45	Tao Ren	peach kernel
90	Zi Ran Ton (dip in vinegar 7 times)	pyrite
60	Tu Bie Chong	wingless cockroach
90	Ma Qian Zi (remove the hairs)	nux vomica seed
90	Xue Jie	dragon's blood resin
30	Jiang Huang	turmeric rhizome
60	Bai Zhi	angelica root
30	Mu Xiang	costus root
30	Chen Pi	ripe tangerine peel
15	Chen Xiang	aloeswood
15	Xiao Hui Xiang	fennel fruit
60	Tian Chi Ginseng	pseudo ginseng
90	Ru Xiang	frankincense
90	Mo Yao	myrrh
90	Chi Shao	red peony
90	Xiang Fu	nut grass rhizome

90	Er Cha	cutch paste
12	Ji Xue Teng	chicken blood vine
30	She Xiang	deer gland secretions
30	Chuan Wu Tou	processed aconite appendage
60	Feng Xian Hua	impatiens flower
60	Ma Huang	hemp yellow
9	Zhu Sha	cinnabar
3	Bing Pian	camphor resin

Analysis of the Herbs in This Formula
Dang Gui enriches the blood and stops pain. Chuan Xiong, Hong Hua, Ji Xue Teng, Tao Ren, and Chi Shao circulate the blood. Zi Ran Ton, Tu Bie Chong, Ru Xiang, Xiao Hui Xiang, She Xiang, and Bing Pian all dissolve blood clots and alleviate pain. Chuan Wu Tou, Mo Yao, and Feng Xian Hua reduce swelling and resolve infection. Tian Chi Ginseng and Xue Jie stop bleeding. Chen Xiang, Jiang Huang, Ma Qian Zi, and Xiang Fu circulate chi. Mu Xiang and Chen Pi calm the stomach. Er Cha clears infection. Zhu Sha has a mild sedative effect. Ma Huang and Bai Zhi accelerate healing.

Recommended Method of Preparation
Mix the herbs and grind them into a fine powder to be made into pills. (See chapter 1 for full instruction on how to make pills.) Traditionally, this formula was prepared as pills; if you prefer, however, you may put the herbs into capsules.

Recommended Dosage
Take 1 to 2 pills (each containing 4.5 grams of powdered herbs) twice daily with room-temperature sweet rice wine until healing is complete.

Caution
Any herbal formula containing Tian Chi Ginseng should not be used by a pregnant woman. It could harm the fetus!

Herbal Oils, Liniments, and Salves

Regular participation in any athletic activity invariably results in occasional injury, and the martial arts are no exception. Admittedly, the potential for serious injury (such as broken bones) does exist to a somewhat greater degree in martial arts than in many other activities, primarily because of the amount of sparring or simulated fighting that is necessary to perfect technique and improve skills. However, when the importance of controlling technique is emphasized, serious injury can be kept to a minimum.

By far the most common injuries seen in martial arts are the minor aches and pains that occur as a result of strenuous daily training. These minor injuries have always been accepted as a normal part of development by martial arts practitioners. Anyone who seriously embarks on the study of martial arts soon becomes familiar with the expression "No pain, no gain."

At one time a standard part of martial arts training was informal instruction in the use of herbal oils and liniments to effectively manage sore muscles and strained ligaments. Such formulas are considered important not only for treating existing injuries but also as a way to avoid any long-range side effects, such as arthritis and rheumatism, that can develop many years after an original injury has occurred.

Herbal Formulas for Oils, Liniments, and Salves

Patent Formulas
Zheng Gu Shui (Rectify Bone Liquid)
Tieh Ta Yao Gin (Traumatic Injury Medicine—Essence)
Hsuing Tan Tieh Wan (Bear Gallbladder Traumatic Injury Pills)
Te Xiao Yao Tong Ling (Specific Lumbaglin)

Zheng Gu Shui Patent Formula

RECTIFY BONE LIQUID

ALSO KNOWN AS ZHENG GU SHUI ANALGESIC LINIMENT

This is without a doubt one of the most powerful liniments available in Chinese medicine. It is especially effective for deep bone bruises and hairline fractures.

When using Zheng Gu Shui special care must be taken by those with fair or delicate skin; prolonged contact can cause blistering or irritation. (If either develops, immediately discontinue use.) However, if you can get past this side effect, this herbal liniment is one of the most effective available.

How to Use This Patent Formula

To properly use Zheng Gu Shui soak a square piece of gauze in the liniment and place it over the injury. Cover the gauze with plastic wrap, making it as airtight as possible. Zheng Gu Shui should start to "heat up" the injured area. Leave it on for 20 to 30 minutes, then remove the gauze and discard.

Caution

Zheng Gu Shui is for external use only. It should not be used on an open wound, cut, or abrasion.

Tieh Ta Yao Gin Patent Formula

TRAUMATIC INJURY MEDICINE—ESSENCE
ALSO KNOWN AS DIE DA YAO JING

While not as powerful as Zheng Gu Shui, Tieh Ta Yao Gin is excellent and can be used for a variety of traumatic injuries. It is effective for treating sprains, torn ligaments, strained muscles, and bruises. It will reduce swelling and repair broken blood vessels; it can be used for cuts and abrasions. It also eliminates dark purple bruised blood and invigorates the chi and blood, thus expediting healing.

Tieh Ta Yao Gin can stain the skin and any clothing that it touches. However, the resulting stain can be wiped off the skin with alcohol or removed from the clothing by washing. Nevertheless, the effectiveness of this formula makes it worthy of your consideration.

How to Use This Patent Formula

Rub this liniment into the injured area, then cover the area with a towel. Keep the towel over the injured area for at least 30 minutes.

HSUING TAN TIEH WAN PATENT FORMULA

BEAR GALLBLADDER TRAUMATIC INJURY PILLS*
ALSO KNOWN AS XIONG DAN DIE DA WAN

Here we have a formula that is very popular in China for the treatment of martial arts injuries. It invigorates blood circulation, reduces swelling, and breaks up stagnant blood while promoting the healing of broken blood vessels. Martial artists use it for all kinds of bruises, sprains, and swelling from the trauma of punches, kicks, falls, and so on.

How to Use This Patent Formula
Hsuing Tan Tieh Wan comes in boxes of 10 pills. Dissolve 1 pill in hot water and drink it like tea. Take a second pill and dissolve it in rubbing alcohol; this should then be rubbed onto the affected area.

Caution
Do not use Hsuing Tan Tieh Wan if there is bleeding or an open wound.

The formula also should not be used internally by a pregnant woman. It could harm the fetus.

* Bear gallbladder is an illegal substance in the United States. See pages 77–78 for more on this subject.

Te Xiao Yao Tong Ling Patent Formula

SPECIFIC LUMBAGLIN

Te Xiao Yao Tong Ling is a famous patent medicine, available in pill form, that is used to relax pulled muscles or tendons and to relieve inflammation. The formula can be used for muscle strain or constriction anywhere in the body. It is excellent for long-term use and can also be considered for use in the early stages of training (for relaxing or warming up muscles and tendons), thereby avoiding some of the soreness and discomfort that normally occur before the body becomes fully conditioned.

How to Use This Patent Medicine
Te Xiao Yao Tong Ling comes in boxes of 24 capsules. Take 1 to 3 capsules daily as needed, according to the instructions included in each package.

Herbal Massage Oils

Among traditional martial artists, the practices of assisting your partner in stretching at the beginning of each training session and of massaging each other at the end of the session were established regimens. It was also customary for the students to massage the master (sensei or sifu). Regular massage was recognized as a valuable tool for preventing injuries, because it maintains the balance and movement of blood and chi.

The use of massage in martial arts dates back many centuries. Ancient martial artists combined therapeutic exercises called Taoist Yoga with massage to prevent and treat injuries as well as certain diseases. Its use was yet another example of Taoist concerns for incorporating the yin-yang principle in all aspects of life—in this case through the passive use of massage (yin) in conjunction with the active movement of martial arts and therapeutic exercise (yang).

At the end of a massage session (especially in cases of injury) a warm compress of Chinese herbs was often used to heighten the effects of the treatment. The following herbal compresses and massage oils were widely used by martial artists; each is famous for its therapeutic effect.

Herbal Massage Oils

Raw Form Preparation
Fang Zhi Gao (Prescription for Herbal Fomentation)

Patent Formulas
Po Sum On Oil (Maintain Peaceful Heart Oil)
Wood Lock Medicated Balm (Chinese Muscle Oil)
Bai Hua You (White Flower Analgesic Oil)

Caution

Massage is contraindicated when:

- There are skin eruptions or rashes
- There are large bruises on the body
- There are varicose veins
- There are tumors or any undiagnosed lumps
- There are cardiovascular problems (such as thrombosis or phlebitis)

Fang Zhi Gao

PRESCRIPTION FOR HERBAL FOMENTATION

At the end of a massage session—especially in cases of injury—a warm compress of Chinese herbs was often used to heighten the effects of the treatment. The herbs in this formula will relax muscles and sinews, invigorate blood circulation, and soothe the tissues. You must prepare the herbal compress using decocted tea.

Preparing and Applying an Herbal Compress

Decoct the herbs as instructed in chapter 1, using the formula shown under "Herbal Ingredients." Let the pot of decocted tea cool down to warm. Have two clean towels ready. Both towels are then immersed in the decocted herb tea. Leave one towel in the tea (to keep it warm) and remove the other, wringing it out until it is damp but not dripping. Spread the warm towel over the area of the body that is to be treated. Be sure the towel is not hot enough to scald the skin. After a 3- to 5-minute interval take out the other towel, wring it dry, and exchange: Put the warm towel on the affected area and the used one back into the decocted herbs to warm again. After 3 to 5 minutes repeat the procedure. Continue doing this 10 or more times in succession. Afterward rub the skin dry and keep the affected area warm.

When conditions permit you can spread 4 to 6 layers of towels over the affected area. The top layer of towels can then be wrapped with oilcloth and covered with a cotton blanket. In this way the heat will not dissipate as quickly. If you are using this multilevel method you can change the towels at longer intervals of 8 to 10 minutes; only 2 or 3 changes will be sufficient.

Herbal Ingredients

GRAMS NEEDED	CHINESE NAME	ENGLISH TRANSLATION
9	Ru Xiang	frankincense
9	Mo Yao	myrrh
9	Chuan Wu Tou	processed aconite appendage
9	Gui Zhi	Saigon cinnamon twig
9	Mu Gua	quince fruit
9	Hong Hua	safflower

Analysis of the Herbs in This Formula

Ru Xiang invigorates blood circulation, while Mo Yao relieves pain and swelling. Chuan Wu Tou and Hong-Hua circulate the blood. Gui Zhi circulates the blood and relaxes muscles and tendons. Mu Gua increases blood circulation, increases chi, and relaxes muscles and tendons.

Recommended Method of Preparation

Make a decoction. (See chapter 1 for instructions.)

Recommended Dosage

Following the instructions given under "Preparing an Herbal Compress," use as much of the decocted tea as needed.

Po Sum On Oil Patent Formula

MAINTAIN PEACEFUL HEART OIL

ALSO KNOWN AS BAO XIN AN YOU

Po Sum On Oil is an excellent massage oil often used by practitioners of *tui na* (Chinese massage) to provide deep therapeutic massage. It is perhaps the best known of the three massage oils mentioned here, and has been around for nearly a century. Not considered a "hot oil," it can be used for general massage but may not be the best choice when there are sprains, pulls, or contusions.

It comes in bottles of either 30 or 100 milliliters.

Wood Lock Medicated Balm

CHINESE MUSCLE OIL PATENT FORMULA

Chinese Muscle Oil, reportedly developed by the renowned Chinese surgeon and inventor of Five Animal Play (Chi Kung) Hua To, is today a generic term for oils commonly used for sore muscles, stiff joints, and muscle spasms. Wood Lock Medicated Balm is one very popular such oil that is also highly regarded as a muscle relaxer. It comes in bottles of 50 milliliters.

Bai Hua You

WHITE FLOWER ANALGESIC OIL PATENT FORMULA

Bai Hua You is an excellent therapeutic massage oil. It is considerably hotter than Po Sum On Oil, and is more effective for use on sore muscles, sprains, strains, and contusions. Bai Hua You comes in small bottles of $1/_3$ ounce.

Caution

Because it contains menthol, camphor, eucalyptus, and lavender oils, take care to avoid getting Bai Hua You in the eyes.

Herbs That Restore Consciousness after Knockout

Perhaps the most serious of all the injuries that can occur during martial arts training is the knockout, or temporary loss of consciousness. It is usually the result of a blow to the head or the uncontrolled application of strangulation technique.

Two formulas mentioned repeatedly in the literature on herbs used by ancient martial artists are said to "arouse the spirit and restore the pulse"—which is traditional Chinese medicine's way of saying "to regain consciousness."

Herbal Formulas That Restore Consciousness After Knockout

Raw Form Preparations
Er Wei Fu Sheng San (Two Flavors Recover Life Powder)
Shaolin Zhen Yu San (Shaolin Precious Jade Powder)

Er Wei Fu Sheng San

TWO FLAVORS RECOVER LIFE POWDER

Er Wei Fu Sheng San is used by blowing the fine powder into the subject's nostril. Use the right nostril for women, the left nostril for men. They may feel nasal pain when they regain consciousness. If so, apply ginger juice* to relieve it.

You may be wondering—as I did when I first encountered this formula—why the left nostril is used for men and the right for women. Unfortunately, my curiosity concerning this somewhat unusual procedure has never been satisfied; this formula does work, however. When I used it on a victim of fainting as a result of hyperventilation during a sparring session, the subject reported that a distinct burning sensation in the nostril caused immediate arousal.

Herbal Ingredients

GRAMS NEEDED	CHINESE NAME	ENGLISH TRANSLATION
30	Ban Xia	half summer
30	Da Huang	rhubarb root

Analysis of the Herbs in This Formula
The herbs Ban Xia and Da Huang both invigorate blood circulation, arouse the senses, and clear heat.

Recommended Method of Preparation
Mix the herbs and grind them into a fine powder.

Recommended Dosage
Blow a pinch into the left nostril of a man or the right nostril of a woman.

---

*Ginger juice is available commercially in Asian food or health food stores, or it can be made by blending scraped gingerroot pieces in a blender (on medium); place the ginger into a small piece of cheesecloth and squeeze out the ginger juice.

Shaolin Zhen Yu San
SHAOLIN PRECIOUS JADE POWDER

Shaolin Zhen Yu San should be used as a follow-up to Er Wei Fu Sheng San.

After someone has regained consciousness, it is quite normal for him to feel confused or have a temporary loss of memory. Shaolin Zhen Yu San will assist in restoring mental clarity.

Herbal Ingredients

GRAMS NEEDED	CHINESE NAME	ENGLISH TRANSLATION
15	Ming Tian Ma	heavenly hemp
15	Fang Feng	guard against wind
15	Nan Xing (stir-fry in ginger juice *)	jack in the pulpit rhizome
15	Bai Zhi	angelica root
3	Bai Fu Zi	white appendage rhizome

Analysis of the Herbs in This Formula

The herbs Ming Tian Ma, Nan Xing, and Bai Fu Zi are all anticonvulsive and useful for dizziness and strokes. Fang Feng and Bai Zhi both relieve headaches.

Recommended Method of Preparation

Mix the herbs and grind them into a fine powder.

Recommended Dosage

Mix .2 to .3 gram of powder with 4 ounces of sweet rice wine or boiled water. Drink it at room temperature.

---

*Ginger juice is available commercially in Asian food stores or health food stores, or it can be made by blending scraped gingerroot in a blender (on medium); place the ginger into a small piece of cheesecloth and squeeze out the ginger juice.

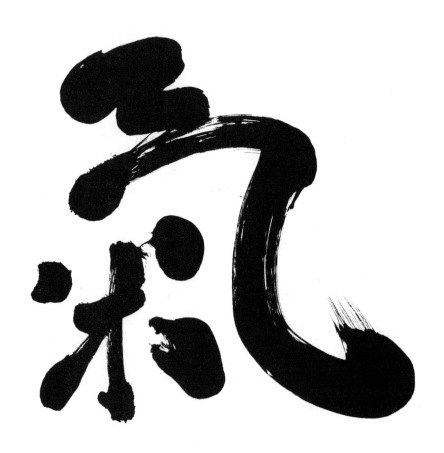

CHI

VITAL ENERGY

3

TRAINING
FORMULAS

In addition to treating injuries common
in the practice of martial arts, herbs were traditionally also used in
what are called training formulas. These formulas are still considered
important by traditional martial artists for developing and maintaining the strength and stamina needed to practice their art. With these
classical training formulas as their foundation, martial artists often
made modifications through trial and error to suit their particular
needs based on the physical demands of certain martial arts styles.
For example, it was not uncommon for practitioners of grasping styles
(like Eagle Claw) or those that use a deep stance (such as Hung Gar)
to add, among other things, bone-strengthening ingredients to the
generic formula. The specific ingredients in these personalized formulas were, as you can imagine, well-guarded secrets!

Unlike injury-management formulas, which are used for occasional sprains, cuts, or contusions, training formulas are used on a
regular basis as a complement to training. Their use appears to demonstrate an awareness of the traditional Chinese medical principle
that states, "Optimum health and a strong physical body depend to a
large extent on maximum organ functioning, which is influenced by
the quality of the chi and blood that supply all of the body's organs
with energy (chi) and nourishment (blood)." The basic function of

training formulas is, therefore, to nourish both chi and blood.

The most common method of consuming training formulas is to drink tea made from herbs. Taken on a regular basis, such teas become an extension of the martial artist's daily nutrition. Indeed, these training formulas are excellent nutritional supplements that you can take regularly for extended periods of time throughout your many years of training.

Tonics for Strengthening the Body and Increasing Stamina

It is only appropriate that the first two formulas I will discuss deal with what traditional Chinese medicine considers the two most primary substances in human physiology—the blood (known as *xue*) and the vital energy (called chi). The powerful influence that the quality of these two substances have on overall health (which is the theoretical basis of traditional Chinese medicine) is emphasized even more in the case of the martial artist, because of the extraordinary physical demands required to practice the art.

Merely describing the blood's main functions—carrying oxygen to the tissues, along with nourishing the vital organs, muscles, skin, tendons, and bones—should leave no doubt concerning its important role in physiology.

While there is little similarity in their basic function, traditional Chinese medicine considers the vital energy and blood equal in terms of their physiological importance. The main function of chi is to supply the energy and stimulation for organ functioning, as well as providing the pep and vigor associated with vibrant health. All physical activity is a manifestation of this vital energy.

Si Wu Tang—which could be considered "the mother of all blood tonics"—is among the most ancient formulas mentioned in Chinese herbal texts, and it is the foundation (containing four basic herbs) on which all other blood tonic formulas are built. It is without a doubt the best known, the most often prescribed, and by many accounts the most effective of all the blood tonic formulas in the Chinese herbal system.

Si Jun Zi Tang could, on the other hand, be considered "the father of all chi tonics," because of the yang or male nature of chi compared to the yin or female nature of the blood. It is also ancient, often prescribed, and effective, along with being the foundation formula (containing four basic herbs) on which many chi tonics are based. It is used extensively in traditional Chinese medicine to restore energy after a long illness or surgery, as well as being used in martial arts for increasing and restoring energy levels whose depletion is a natural result of training.

As I mentioned earlier and will note again in the following training formulas, Shih Chuang Da Bu Wan, Tai Chi Tea, Huang Ti Tang, and Jin Gu Jia Wan are all based upon these two foundation formulas. It can not be overemphasized that the herbs that make up Si Wu Tang and Si Jun Zi Tang are among the most important and frequently used herbs in the Chinese herbal system. One or the other is the main ingredient in some of the most powerful tonic formulas in Chinese herbology. Anyone with even a casual interest in Chinese herbology would be well advised to become familiar with them.

Tonic Formulas for Strengthening the Body and Increasing Stamina

Raw Form Preparations
Si Wu Tang (Four-Substance Decoction)
Si Jun Zi Tang (Four-Gentlemen Decoction)
Tai Chi Tea (All-Inclusive Great Tonifying Decoction)
Huang Ti Tang (Double Harmony Tea)
Jin Gu Jia Wan (Golden Relics Pills)

Patent Formulas
Shih Chuan Da Bu Wan (All-Inclusive Great Tonifying Pills)

Si Wu Tang

FOUR-SUBSTANCE DECOCTION

This formula is noted for its ability to enrich, regulate, and circulate the blood. It is without a doubt the most famous blood tonic in Chinese herbology.

Anemia and poor circulation are disharmonies of the blood associated with fatigue (anemia) and lack of flexibility (poor circulation). By enriching the blood anemia is avoided, by regulating it all of the organs benefit, and by circulating the blood flexibility and movement of the joints are improved.

Herbal Ingredient

GRAMS NEEDED	CHINESE NAME	ENGLISH TRANSLATION
3	Dang Gui	tang-kuei root
3	Bai Shao	white peony root
3	Chuan Xiong	lovage root
3	Shu Di Huang	wine-cooked Chinese foxglove root

Analysis of the Herbs in This Formula

Dang Gui enriches the blood and stops pain, Bai Shao also enriches the blood, Chuan Xiong circulates the blood, and Shu Di Huang nourishes the blood and regulates the blood flow.

Recommended Method of Preparation

Make a decoction. (See chapter 1 for instructions.)

Recommended Dosage

Drink 4 ounces of Si Wu Tang tea at room temperature 3 times daily, or 6 ounces twice daily.

Si Jun Zi Tang
FOUR-GENTLEMEN DECOCTION

Si Jun Zi Tang is an ancient, classical formula useful for supplementing and restoring the energy that is lost through training.

Herbal Ingredients

GRAMS NEEDED	CHINESE NAME	ENGLISH TRANSLATION
3	Ren Shen	ginseng root
3	Bai Zhu	atractylodis rhizome
3	Fu Ling	tuckahoe root
1	Zhu Gan Cao	honey-cooked licorice

Analysis of the Herbs in This Formula

Ren Shen (ginseng) increases the chi. Bai Zhu, in addition to increasing the vital energy, strengthens the immune system. Fu Ling strengthens the spleen and stomach. Zhu Gan Cao increases the chi and harmonizes (improves the taste of) the other herbs in the formula.

Recommended Method of Preparation

Prepare a decoction or medicinal wine. (See chapter 1 for instructions.)

Recommended Dosage

For herbs used in a decoction, drink 4 ounces of Si Jun Zi Tang tea at room temperature 3 times daily, or 6 ounces 2 times daily. For herbs used in a medicinal wine, drink 1 ounce daily at room temperature or mix 1 ounce of medicinal wine with 3 ounces of tepid water and drink once daily.

Tai Chi Tea

ALL-INCLUSIVE GREAT TONIFYING DECOCTION
ALSO KNOWN AS SHI QUAN DA BU TANG OR SHIH
CHUAN DA BU TANG

Tai Chi Tea is an example of a major training formula in which you will find all eight of the herbs in the two previous formulas. Originally known as Ten Complete Great Invigorating Herbs Tea, this centuries-old training formula tonifies the blood and the chi and is commonly used by martial artists for improving overall health while increasing vitality. Tai Chi Tea is especially useful for promoting endurance and speeding recovery after a strenuous training session.

Herbal Ingredients

GRAMS NEEDED	CHINESE NAME	ENGLISH TRANSLATION
3	Ren Shen	ginseng root
3	Bai Zhu	atractylodis rhizome
1	Zhu Gan Cao	honey-cooked licorice
3	Fu Ling	tuckahoe root
3	Shu Di Huang	wine-cooked Chinese foxglove root
3	Chuan Xiong	lovage root
3	Dang Gui	tang-kuei root
3	Bai Shao	white peony root
3	Huang Qi	milk vetch root
3	Rou Gui	cinnamon bark

Analysis of the Herbs in This Formula

Ren Shen (ginseng) increases the chi, while Bai Zhu increases energy and strengthens immunity. Zhu Gan Cao increases the vital energy and improves the formula's flavor. Fu Ling strengthens the spleen and stomach. Shu Di Huang enriches the blood. Dang Gui and Bai Shao assist in nourishing the blood, while Chuan Xiong circulates it. Huang Qi increases vital energy, builds the immune system, and strengthens the lungs (which is especially good for

Chi Kung and Tai Chi). Rou Gui increases the vital energy and strengthens the spleen and kidneys.

Recommended Method of Preparation
Make a decoction or medicinal wine. (See chapter 1 for instructions.)

Recommended Dosage
For herbs used in a decoction, drink 4 ounces of Tai Chi Tea at room temperature 3 times daily, or drink 6 ounces twice daily. For herbs used in a medicinal wine, drink 1 ounce daily at room temperature or mix 1 ounce of medicinal wine with 3 ounces of tepid water and drink once daily.

Tai Chi Tea is also available in a prepared patent form called Shih Chuan Da Bu Wan—Ten Flavor Tea (All-Inclusive Great Tonifying Pills). It comes in bottles of 200 pills with instructions for recommended dosage included. This same formula is also available under the name Shih Chuan Ta Bu Wan (All-Inclusive Great Tonifying Pills) and comes in bottles of 120 pills.

HUANG TI TANG

DOUBLE HARMONY TEA

Ancient texts make frequent mention of the Yellow Emperor Huang Ti's considerable skill in the art of classical Chinese wrestling. It is also common knowledge that the emperor enlisted the help of Taoist priests to conduct experiments in his search for immortality. Any Taoist prescription for life extension would have undoubtedly included some form of therapeutic exercise, meditation, and herbal therapy.

This particular formula is reputed to have been Emperor Huang Ti's preferred herbal preparation. It is aptly named considering its mild, balanced nature. Huang Ti Tang (Double Harmony Tea) will nourish both blood and chi and can be used effectively for extended periods of time to treat exhaustion, or what might be called burnout, due to overtraining.

Herbal Ingredients

GRAMS NEEDED	CHINESE NAME	ENGLISH TRANSLATION
2	Dang Gui	tang-kuei root
2	Shu Di Huang	wine-cooked Chinese foxglove root
5	Bai Shao	white peony root
2	Chuan Xiong	lovage root
2	Huang Qi	milk vetch root
1	Zhu Gan Cao	honey-cooked licorice
1	Sheng Jiang	ginger rhizome
1	Da Zao	jujube fruit
1	Rou Gui	cinnamon bark

Analysis of the Herbs in This Formula

Dang Gui, Shu Di Huang, and Bai Shao nourish the blood, while Chuan Xiong circulates it. Huang Qi increases chi and strengthens the immune system and lungs. Zhu Gan Cao increases vital energy and improves the taste of the formula. Sheng Jiang harmonizes the spleen and stomach, while Da Zao nourishes the blood and moderates the action of the other herbs in the formula. Rou Gui increases the vital energy and strengthens the kidneys and spleen.

Recommended Method of Preparation
Prepare a decoction or medicinal wine. (See chapter 1 for instructions.)

Recommended Dosage
For herbs used in a decoction, drink 4 ounces of Huang Ti Tang at room temperature 3 times daily. For herbs used in a medicinal wine, drink 1 ounce daily at room temperature or mix 1 ounce with 3 ounces of tepid water and drink once daily.

JIN GU JIA WAN

GOLDEN RELICS PILLS

Another important formula in Chinese herbology that is useful to
martial artists is Jin Gu Jia Wan, which nourishes the body's vital
fluids while supporting hormone levels and tonifying the blood.
The ability of Jin Gu Jia Wan to nourish all of the body's fluids,
including the synovial fluid (which lubricates the joints), is the
main reason that this formula was so widely used by ancient
martial artists who suffered problems with flexibility and creaking
joints.

It is important to note that the flexibility prerequisite for all
styles of martial arts practice should not be overlooked in favor of
developing what is often called a muscle-bound physique. I highly
recommend this formula for use by all martial artists for improving
flexibility.

To avoid confusion, it should be pointed out that this is a raw
herb formula that must be decocted into tea, despite the fact that
its name implies otherwise. Unfortunately, this formula cannot be
prepared in pill form.

Herbal Ingredients

GRAMS NEEDED	CHINESE NAME	ENGLISH TRANSLATION
3	Shu Di Huang	wine-cooked Chinese foxglove root
2	Shan Zhu Yu	dried cornelian cherry
2	Shan Yao	Chinese yam root
1.5	Mu Dan Pi	peony root bark
1.5	Fu Ling	tuckahoe root
1.5	Ze Xie	water plantain
1.5	Niu Xi	ox-knee root
1.5	Che Qian Zi	plantago seed
1.5	Gou Qi Zi	matrimony fruit

Analysis of the Herbs in This Formula

Shu Di Huang enriches the blood. Shan Zhu Yu and Shan Yao act together to strengthen the liver, kidneys, and spleen while also strengthening the knees. Mu Dan Pi increases blood circulation. Fu Ling strengthens the spleen and stomach. Ze Xie affects fluids in the lower body, and Niu Xi treats weakness in the lower limbs. Che Qian Zi and Gou Qi Zi strengthen the liver and kidneys and increase yin fluids.

Recommended Method of Preparation
Prepare a decoction. (See chapter 1 for instructions.)

Recommended Dosage
Drink 4 ounces of room-temperature tea 3 times daily.

Medicinal Wines That Strengthen the Body and Increase Stamina

Although the training formulas in this section have distinctly different applications, what they have in common is their recommended method of preparation—aging herbs in alcohol to create medicinal wines (or Jui Dan). Instructions for preparing medicinal wine can be found in chapter 1.

Medicinal Wine Formulas Used to Strengthen the Body and Increase Stamina

Raw Form Preparation

Hu Gu Ren Shen Jiu (Tiger Bone Ginseng Liquor)*
Lu Rong Ren Shen Jiu (Deer Antler Ginseng Liquor)
Chun Jiu (Spring Wine—Seasonal Wine)
Dong Chou Jiu (Winter Training Wine—Seasonal Wine)

---

* Tiger bone is an illegal substance in the United States. See pages 77–78 for more on this subject.

Hu Gu Ren Shen Jiu

TIGER BONE GINSENG LIQUOR

Both this formula and the one that follows, Lu Rong Ren Shen Jiu, powerfully tonify the vital energy as well as strengthening the bones, joints, and lower back. The difference between the two is that Hu Gu Ren Shen Jiu acts more specifically to strengthen the bones and joints, and increase the bone density. Lu Rong Ren Shen Jiu has a stronger effect on increasing testosterone levels; its bone-strengthening capabilities are minor in comparison. The increased sexual energy that is the result can further benefit energy levels, or it can be useful in the Taoist sexual practices I discuss in chapter 4.

When prepared with high-quality ingredients and properly aged these medicinal wines are among the most potent herbal elixirs available, and are well worth the effort involved in preparing them. There are, however, several drawbacks. The first is that selling tiger bone is illegal—although it is available under the counter in Chinatowns across the United States (especially those on the East and West Coasts). Second is that the cost of tiger bone, fresh deer antler, and high-quality ginseng—all considered "precious ingredients"—can be extremely high.

Over the centuries tiger bone, which has a well-known reputation for strengthening bones, joints, and ligaments, has often been the main ingredient in formulas used in traditional Chinese medicine to treat diseases affecting the bones and joints (such as arthritis, osteoporosis, and spondylitis). Because of these abilities to strengthen bones and joints, especially those of the lower body, Hu Gu Ren Shen Jiu is particularly valuable to martial artists who practice styles that use a deep stance, as well as those who practice standing meditation.

The near extinction of the tiger has in recent years created diminishing supplies of tiger bone, which has resulted in many substitutes being sold, including leopard, horse, and canine bones. All have proven inferior in terms of their strength and overall effect compared with the results seen with tiger bone.

I should also mention that there are some moral issues you must consider when using tiger bone. As a martial artist who has used herbs over the past twenty years, and the owner of a mail-order Chinese herb company (Treasures from the Sea of Chi), I have personally struggled with this issue and have come to the decision that even though animal organs and by-products are a legitimate part of the five-thousand-year-old Chinese herbal system, my conscience will not allow me to use any product that requires the killing or harming of any animal. I will, however, leave this decision strictly up to each individual.

Herbal Ingredients

GRAMS NEEDED	CHINESE NAME	ENGLISH TRANSLATION
10	Ren Shen	ginseng root
10	Hu Gu	tiger bone

Analysis of the Herbs in This Formula
Hu Gu strengthens the sinews and bones, and it is useful for pain and weakness in the knees and lower back as well as stiffness in the joints. Ren Shen will powerfully increase the chi, and the alcohol will invigorate the blood.

Recommended Method of Preparation
Grind the herbs into a fine powder and make a medicinal wine. (See chapter 1 for instructions.)

Recommended Dosage
Drink 1 ounce of room-temperature wine daily. This formula can be safely taken for extended periods of time throughout your years of training.

Lu Rong Ren Shen Jiu

DEER ANTLER GINSENG LIQUOR

For reasons unknown to me deer antler (Lu Rong) lacks the notoriety of herbs like ginseng, except among knowledgeable herb users, even though it is reputed to have a more powerful effect on sexual functioning than ginseng (which works more specifically to increase energy levels). Widely used for sexual enhancement and dysfunction, deer antler increases chi, improves immunity, raises testosterone levels, and strengthens the bones and sinews.

The quality of this particular ingredient is very important if you are to realize your desired effects. Although Lu Rong is available and sold year-round in Chinese herb stores, knowledgeable users purchase it during the rutting or mating season, when it is freshest and the deer's hormones are at maximum levels. Tender new velvet horn with dried blood still in the cartilage is considered high quality. I should mention that deer antler can be used in good conscience, because (unlike tiger bone) it is harvested without injuring the animal.

When you pay attention to these details and use high-quality deer horn and ginseng, the resulting Lu Rong Ren Shen Jiu is powerful in its effects.

Herbal Ingredients

GRAMS NEEDED	CHINESE NAME	ENGLISH TRANSLATION
10	Lu Rong	deer antler
10	Ren Shen	ginseng root

Analysis of the Herbs in This Formula

Lu Rong strengthens the sinews and bones, benefits the essence (increases testosterone levels), and strengthens the liver and kidneys. Ren Shen will increase chi levels, and alcohol will invigorate the blood.

Recommended Method of Preparation
Grind the herbs into a fine powder, then prepare a medicinal wine. (See chapter 1 for instructions.)

Recommended Dosage
Drink 1 ounce of medicinal wine at room temperature daily. This formula can be safely taken for extended periods of time throughout your years of training.

Seasonal Wines—
Spring and Winter Wines

The first thing you are likely to notice about seasonal wine formulas is the large number of ingredients in them. These all-purpose tonics contain individual ingredients that are specific in their ability to strengthen (tonify) all five of the major organs: lungs, liver, kidneys, heart, and spleen. Additionally, seasonal wines contain ingredients that increase vital energy and nourish the blood, along with herbs that effectively regulate internal body temperatures to correspond with external climatic conditions.

In other words, seasonal wines are most effective when they are used during the season for which they are named. For example Chun Jiu (spring wine), which contains herbs with internal cooling qualities, should be used during the warmer months, while Dong Chou Jiu (winter training wine), which contains herbs that warm the interior body, is most effective during the colder seasons.

It is customary to cure seasonal wines for an entire year. A Chun Jiu, for instance, is made in the spring for consumption the following spring.

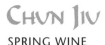

CHUN JIU

SPRING WINE

This potent training formula will nourish the chi, the blood, and the essence. Its ability to nourish the yin body fluids produces a cooling effect on the internal body temperature, which is most effective when used during the warm-weather months (late spring to early autumn).

Herbal Ingredients

GRAMS NEEDED	CHINESE NAME	ENGLISH TRANSLATION
25	Lu Rong	deer antler
25	Lu Jiao Jiao	deer antler glue
25	E Jiao	donkey skin glue
10	Dang Gui	tang-kuei root
25	Shu Di Huang	wine-cooked Chinese foxglove root
12	Huang Qi	milk vetch root
4	Ren Shen	ginseng root
10	Nu Zhen Zi	privet fruit
4	Fu Pen Zi	Chinese raspberry fruit
10	Gou Qi Zi	matrimony fruit
10	Zi He Che	human placenta
10	Hai Ma	sea horse
10	Suo Yang	lock yang stem

PLUS

1 whole piece Ge Jie (gecko lizard)

Analysis of the Herbs in This Formula

Lu Rong strengthens bones and sinews, benefits the essence (increases testosterone levels), and strengthens the liver and kidneys. Lu Jian Jiao strengthens the function of the Lu Rong. E Jiao, Dang Gui, and Shu Di Huang all nourish and enrich the blood. Huang Qi increases chi and strengthens the immune system as well as the lungs. Ren Shen increases vital energy. Nu Zhen Zi and Fu Pen Zi strengthen the liver and kidneys. Gou Qi Zi also strengthens the liver and kidneys, and nourishes the yin fluids. Zi He Che increases vital energy and blood, in addition to strengthening the heart, lungs, and kidneys. Hai Ma improves blood circulation and strengthens the kidneys. Suo Yang nourishes the sexual function and strengthens muscles and bones. Ge Jie strengthens the lungs and kidneys.

Recommended Method of Preparation

You can grind the herbs into a fine powder or use them whole to make a medicinal wine. (See chapter 1 for instructions.) Age this wine for 12 months—for example, from one spring until the following spring.

Recommended Dosage

Drink 1 ounce of medicinal wine at room temperature daily. This formula can be safely taken for extended periods of time, but limit its use to the period from late spring to early autumn.

DONG CHOU JIU

WINTER TRAINING WINE

Dong Chou Jiu will nourish and warm the body while improving the circulation of the blood and chi. It will also strengthen the bones and build up the immune system to ward off perverse energies. This formula is best used during the fall and winter seasons (late autumn to early spring).

Herbal Ingredients

GRAMS NEEDED	CHINESE NAME	ENGLISH TRANSLATION
25	Hu Gu	tiger bone*
25	Lu Rong	deer antler
4	Ren Shen	ginseng root
3	Wu Jia Pi	five-bark root
6	Dang Gui	tang-kuei root
3	Niu Xi	ox-knee root
3	Gou Qi Zi	matrimony fruit
3	Du Zhong	eucommia bark
3	Mu Gua	quince fruit

Analysis of Herbs in This Formula

Hu Gu strengthens the sinews and bones, as well as the knees and lower back, and eliminates stiffness in knees and joints. Lu Rong supports the strengthening of sinews and bones, increases testosterone levels, and strengthens the liver and kidneys. Combined, these two herbs are very warm and dry. Ren Shen increases vital energy. Wu Jia Pi also strengthens the bones and sinews. Dang Gui enriches the blood. Niu Xi, Du Zhong, and Mu Gua strengthen the bones and muscles, treat weak knees, and improve circulation. Gou Qi Zi strengthens the liver and kidneys and nourishes the fluids.

* Tiger bone is an illegal substance in the United States. See pages 77–78 for more on this subject.

Recommended Method of Preparation
You can grind the herbs down into a powder or use them whole to make a medicinal wine. (See chapter 1 for instructions.) Age this wine for 12 months—for example, from one winter to the following winter.

Recommended Dosage
Drink 1 ounce of medicinal wine at room temperature daily. This formula can be safely taken for extended periods of time, but limit its use to the period from late autumn to early spring.

Chinese Herbal Liniments Used for Hand Conditioning

It is not unreasonable to assume that any sport in which you use your hands as striking weapons (such as boxing, the martial arts, or even basic self-defense) would require a certain amount of hand conditioning in order to avoid injury. In this section I will discuss some general guidelines as well as herbal formulas that you can use to safely toughen and condition your hands.

The guidelines I am referring to are basic concepts common to all martial arts styles, which have been handed down from teacher to student for countless generations. Within these principles there are several important points to consider. First, I must emphasize the importance of using herbal liniments to repair damage and avoid any permanent injury. Second, exercise prudence in the amount of training you undertake. Finally, never forget the wisdom of proceeding slowly.

Although they are few in number and for the most part little known, some martial arts styles still use centuries-old secret hand-conditioning formulas that the styles' originators developed. These are, however, the exception to the rule. The vast majority of martial artists must depend on generic, all-purpose liniments to condition their bodies' striking surfaces.

Generally speaking, two basic types of liniments are used—hot and cold. Hot liniments that contain warming herbs are used in both the beginning and intermediate phases of development, known as the yang external stage, while cold liniments that contain cooling herbs are reserved for use in the third and final phase of conditioning, or the yin internal stage.

Typically, the herbs used in hot liniments relax the ligaments and tendons; they also prevent blood clotting and bruising by improving the circulation of the blood and chi. Ingredients in cold liniments gather the chi as they harden and strengthen the bones.

Herbal Formulas for Hand Conditioning

Raw Form Preparations

Fang Sou Yi (Formula Number One)
Du Fang Sou Er (Ministerial Formula Number Two)
Fang Sou San (Formula Number Three)

Fang Sou Yi

FORMULA NUMBER ONE

Fang Sou Yi is an all-purpose hot liniment that you can use in the initial stage of training to condition any of your body's striking surfaces (fists, forearms, shins, and so on).

Herbal Ingredients

GRAMS NEEDED	CHINESE NAME	ENGLISH TRANSLATION
6	Tian Chi Ginseng	pseudo ginseng root
9	Zhang Nao	camphor
9	Bo He	peppermint
6	Yu Jin	turmeric tuber
3	She Xiang	deer gland secretions
6	Dang Gui	tang-kuei root
9	Bing Pian	camphor resin

Analysis of the Herbs in This Formula

Tian Chi Ginseng stops bleeding. Zhang Nao is anti-inflammatory and analgesic. Bo He opens the pores of the skin. Yu Jin prevents blood clotting and relieves pain. She Xiang circulates the blood and prevents inflammation. Dang Gui enriches blood. Bing Pian relieves pain.

Recommended Method of Preparation

Mix the herbs and grind them into a fine powder, then prepare a medicinal wine by curing the herbs in a fifth of brandy. (See chapter 1 for instructions on how to prepare a medicinal wine.) If price is a consideration, alcohol (ethanol) can be substituted for the brandy. Once this medicinal wine has been properly aged, it should be used as a liniment—do not use internally!

Recommended Dosage and Use

The proper way to use an herbal liniment is to massage it into the hands before and after striking practice. Upon application, you will feel a warm tingling sensation accompanied by a reddening of the skin. After approximately 6 to 12 months of use, depending on your diligence in using the liniment, you will experience a lessening of the tingling sensation.

Caution
This formula is for external use only!

When you no longer feel the tingling, this indicates that you have progressed to the next level of training and should change to the next formula, Du Fang Sou Er (Ministerial Formula Number Two), which is hotter than this one.

Du Fang Sou Er

MINISTERIAL FORMULA NUMBER TWO

Before I discuss the ingredients in this liniment, I will take a minute to explain what *ministerial* means. In Chinese herbology this term refers to herbs or formulas that contain certain toxic substances that make their prolonged use prohibitive. Therefore, a word of caution is always given concerning the hazards of inappropriate use.

The important points to remember for safely using a ministerial formula are:

- Limit use to no longer than 90 days
- Use only after completing the initial yang external stage of training
- Use only on the hands; avoid use on the other striking areas of the body

After you use this formula for approximately 90 days, you will see a noticeable difference in the texture of your skin. You will also notice an increased tolerance for striking without bruising or lacerating the striking surface. This is the intermediate stage of development—what is sometimes referred to as "heavy hands." As your hands become more conditioned and you develop speed and good technique (proper use of the hips), the quality of your punches and strikes will progressively increase.

Herbal Ingredients

GRAMS NEEDED	CHINESE NAME	ENGLISH TRANSLATION
6	Bo He	peppermint
3	Fu Zi	aconite root
6	Bi Ba	long pepper fruit
6	Zhang Nao	camphor
6	Ding Xiang	clove flower bud
6	Bai Dou Kou	cardamom

PLUS

> 1 ounce cayenne tincture
> 1 ounce cassia oil
> 1 ounce mineral oil
> 1 ounce lavender oil
> 1 ounce cajeput oil
> 1 ounce olive oil
> 1 ounce eucalyptus oil

Analysis of the Herbs in This Formula

Bo He opens the pores, Fu Zi relieves pain, and Bi Ba is analgesic. Zhang Nao is also analgesic as well as anti-inflammatory. Ding Xiang is antibacterial, and Bai Dou Kou promotes circulation of the energy in the hands. Cayenne tincture is hot; it opens the pores and circulates the blood. Cassia oil is neutral and prevents abrasions; mineral oil is neutral and prevents scarring and abrasions; lavender oil is warm, fragrant, and soothing; cajeput oil is neutral and circulates the blood; olive oil is neutral and binds the other oils together; and, finally, eucalyptus oil is cool and will soothe the skin surface.

Recommended Method of Preparation

Mix the Chinese herbs and grind them into a fine powder. You can locate the cayenne tincture and the oils at a health food store or order from one of the catalogs mentioned in appendix 4.

Then prepare a medicinal wine by curing the herbs and oils in rectified turpentine. (Rectified turpentine is refined or purified turpentine that is used medicinally, and it can be found in health food stores and pharmacies or in mail-order catalogs.) In a 1-liter glass container, mix the ground herbs, tincture, and oils, then top off the container with the turpentine. (See chapter 1 for exact instructions.) Once this mixture has been properly aged it should be used only as a liniment—do not use internally!

Recommended Dosage and Use

The proper way to use this ministerial formula is to massage the liniment into the hands before and after striking practice. Limit use to no longer than 90 days.

Caution
This formula is for external use only!

―――――――――

This outer or external conditioning formula concludes the yang external stage of training. We are now ready to turn our attention to hardening and strengthening the underlying internal structures (bones) in the final yin internal stage.

FANG SOU SAN
FORMULA NUMBER THREE

As you might expect, massaging this next cold liniment, Fang Sou San, into the hands produces a cold sensation that you will feel in your fingers as well. Unlike the previous formula, Du Fang Sou Er, whose use is restricted to no more than 90 days, you can use this final hand-conditioning formula for longer periods without experiencing any deleterious effects.

Normally, you will use this formula (like Fang Sou Yi) for 6 to 12 months before completing the final yin internal stage of training. When you no longer experience a cold sensation after applying the liniment, it is an indication that the hand-conditioning process has been completed.

Remember that excellent technique and brilliant strategy are of little use if your primary weapons—your hands—are injured. The hand-conditioning process is important for all Chinese, Japanese, and Korean boxing styles. Beyond the use of liniments and the three developmental stages, hand conditioning is a continuous process using methods such as heavy bag training, Makawara striking, knuckle push-ups, and the 108 movements of the "Wooden Man."

Herbal Ingredients

GRAMS NEEDED	CHINESE NAME	ENGLISH TRANSLATION
3	Gua Lou	heavenly flower fruit
6	Bo He	peppermint
3	Bai Zhi	angelica root
6	Huang Lian	golden thread
3	Xiang Fu	nut grass rhizome

PLUS

3 ounces peppermint oil
3 ounces eucalyptus oil

Analysis of the Herbs in This Formula
Gua Lou promotes healing, Bo He opens the pores, and Bai Zhi

reduces swelling. Huang Lian reduces inflammation, and Xiang Fu reduces pain and circulates chi in the hands. Peppermint and eucalyptus oils are cool and will soothe the skin surface; combined they have a stronger effect soothing the skin and bones.

Recommended Method of Preparation

Mix the Chinese herbs and grind them into a fine powder. You can locate the oils at a health food store or in one of the mail-order catalogs listed in appendix 4. Then prepare a medicinal wine by curing the herbs and oils in equal parts of alcohol (ethanol) and rectified turpentine. (Rectified turpentine is refined or purified turpentine that is used medicinally; you can find it in health food stores and pharmacies or in the mail-order catalogs listed in the appendix.) In a 1-liter glass container mix the ground herbs and oils, then top off the container with equal parts of alcohol and turpentine. (See chapter 1 for exact instructions.) Once this mixture has been properly aged, it should be used only as a liniment—do not use internally!

Recommended Dosage and Use

Massage the cold liniment into your hands before and after striking practice until you no longer feel a cold sensation after applying.

Caution

This formula is for external use only!

Before closing out this section, I would like to offer some reassurance to those who might be overly concerned about the possibility of serious injury. When you follow the basic guidelines for hand conditioning there is very little likelihood of injury occurring. If, however, you find yourself among the small percentage of martial artists who are unfortunate enough to sustain an injury during the hand-conditioning process, immediately suspend your training and use the appropriate formula (which you can find in chapter 2: "Injury-Management Formulas")—but only as an adjunct to treatment by a qualified physician.

Ginseng

No reference work on Chinese herbology would be complete without a discussion of the most controversial, well-known, and misused of all Chinese herbs—ginseng. Although it is available in many different forms, including teas, tinctures, and pills, misinformation concerning proper dosage and the length of time that it should be taken—and, perhaps most important, the inability to choose high-quality ginseng due to lack of experience—have resulted in wide-scale improper use of this legendary herb.

Consequently, most users have not truly experienced ginseng's powerful tonifying effects and wrongfully assume its reputation is unfounded. Ginseng's power should not be underestimated!

On the following pages I will give some guidelines for the proper use of ginseng by anyone interested in using what is considered "the greatest of all Chinese tonic herbs." This information is meant to be applied when ginseng is used as a single herb, not as part of a formula.

On all levels of training—from beginning (white belt) to advanced (black belt)—and regardless of the style of martial arts that is being practiced, great emphasis is placed on the importance of developing the body's vital energy. Whether this vital energy is referred to as chi in Chinese Kung Fu, *qi* in Japanese Karate, or *ki* in Korean Tae Kwon Do, it is one and the same.

Theoretically speaking, three components are needed to cultivate and develop chi:

- The particular kind of abdominal breathing that is the foundation of Chinese Kung Fu (Dan Tien), as well as Japanese and Korean disciplines (*hara* breathing)
- The practice of sexual conservation, or limiting the loss of sexual energy and fluids (semen) through sex
- The alteration of the vibratory rate, which is accomplished through meditation

Additionally, the use of herbs can also be effective in increasing energy levels. Of all of the herbal plant medicines, ginseng is unquestionably the most powerful for effectively increasing the body's vital energy.

In order to experience the extraordinary tonifying capabilities of ginseng, you must take these three points into consideration:

- The quality of the root
- The dosage or amount you take
- The length of time you take the ginseng

Since ginseng's introduction to the Western world by Jesuit priests in the late seventeenth century, the high price of this herb has created a great temptation for unscrupulous merchants to adulterate it with other substances and misrepresent its quality to uninformed consumers. Regrettably, these deceptive practices continue today. Because of this, I advise you to restrict your use to raw ginseng root, avoiding teas, pills, and capsules.

The exorbitant price of ginseng can be somewhat justified by the stringent requirements of its cultivation. Growing a plant from seed to maturity requires a minimum seven-year wait before it can be harvested. Not surprisingly, due to supply and demand many roots are harvested prematurely, and poor-quality roots end up proliferating the ginseng market.

The quality of ginseng is determined by three factors:

- Its age (the older it is, the more potent)
- Where it's grown
- Whether it is grown wild or cultivated

The highest-quality, and most expensive, ginseng available is Manchurian ginseng that has been grown wild for seven years or longer. Korean and Chinese ginsengs are both excellent, but of lower quality. The most readily available ginseng is cultivated Korean (red) and Chinese (shi chu) ginseng. These are normally three to six years old, moderately priced, and account for approximately 90 percent of the ginseng on the market.

It cannot be overstated that the supply of wild ginseng (Korean, Chinese, and especially Manchurian) is extremely limited. Unless you are certain about the integrity of the source from which you are purchasing it—buyer, beware!

I should also mention that the raw root, which is sold by the single root or by the catty (1¹/₂ pounds), does not include instructions on dosage.

Another stumbling block toward use is the variation in quality that can make it difficult to determine effective dosage. Therefore, each person needs to experiment to find the dosage that works best. Generally speaking, you can best be guided by the traditional Chinese recommendation: 1 gram of steamed ginseng root chewed 2 to 3 times daily for at least a month. The longer you take it and the higher its quality, the more powerful are its effects.

It is also interesting to note that people with moderately vegetarian or macrobiotic diets usually notice the effects of ginseng sooner than those who indulge in rich, highly spiced meat diets.

Here in the West, ginseng's fame has developed because of its reputation for increasing virility and enhancing sexual abilities. Although there is some truth to these claims, preoccupation with its reported sexual benefits has created confusion about its main function.

What makes ginseng of such great value to martial artists is its often-overlooked ability to increase energy levels. Additionally, ginseng users report increases in physical strength and stamina as well as improved reflexes. All of these positive effects are not only valuable in the practice of the martial arts but also important elements of good health in general.

They can be virtually guaranteed if the recommended dosage, time frame, and quality of ginseng are not compromised.

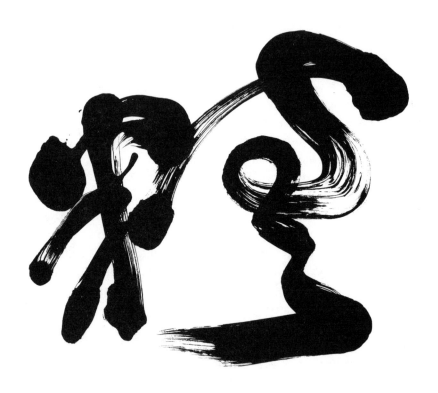

JING

SEXUAL ENERGY

4

Herbs for the

Taoist Practice

of Sexual

Conservation

No one can say with any degree of certainty where or when the practice of sexual conservation, known as *liu fang ching*, began. Even though it is associated with Taoism (which causes many to falsely assume that this is where it originated), it has always been one of the primary disciplines of mysticism and is not exclusive to any particular culture or religion.

This ancient practice, which is among the highest religious doctrines, is practiced by clerical members of some of the major religions mainly because of its role in spiritual development. Priestly celibacy is probably the most familiar example of it. In addition to claims of nurturing the spirit, sexual conservation has been credited with contributing to extraordinary feats of strength as well as enhancing overall mental clarity.

Supporters of the theories on regulating or conserving sex insist that the U.S. military's attempt to subordinate the sexual urge during basic training, by separating women and men and the controversial use of sexual suppressants (saltpeter) in food, validates these claims.

Further evidence of the application of this theory can be seen in many forms of athletics. For example, the practice of discouraging sex by banning women from the training camps of professional boxers and football coaches' attempts to enforce temporary abstinence among team members before a game are both based on the theory of sexual conservation and the role that it plays in increasing strength and endurance, as well as improving the mental focus of athletic participants.

Since the martial arts are essentially forms of athletics, it should come as no surprise that the practice of conserving sexual energy is an integral part of the esoteric study of martial arts known as Shen Kung, which is more commonly referred to as "storing the essence and circulating the chi."

One hundred days of sexual abstinence is the time frame that is usually recommended to Shen Kung practitioners in order to increase the chi to levels that allow them to circulate it and experience the psychic and physical phenomena that result from this sexual-alchemical process.

Admittedly, the self-control required for this is difficult, but it is by no means impossible. First and foremost we must employ what my martial arts teacher and mentor Shidoshi Ron Van Clief refers to as "iron will." We are also fortunate to have at our disposal herbal remedies that can assist us in controlling the loss of seminal fluids.

Because of our tendency toward overindulgence, it may quite often be necessary to replenish the sexual energy before the practice of Shen Kung can begin in earnest. In this chapter I offer several herbal formulas to help you reestablish functional sexual energy levels.

For those who want to continue to have sex but avoid ejaculation in order to practice Shen Kung, I also include a formula that is commonly used in Taoist sex practice.

The debate surrounding the efficacy of the practice of sexual conservation will undoubtedly persist. It has been and always will be a source of controversy. However, most people who arbitrarily dismiss it and its reported powerful effects usually do so because of their own inability to free themselves from the sensory enslavement to sex that is a constant deterrent to fully realizing human potential. Martial artists who are interested in reaching the highest levels of training by developing the body, mind, and spirit should find such practice, and the following herbal formulas, helpful.

Herbal Formulas Used for the Taoist Practice of Sexual Conservation

Raw Form Preparations

Jin Feng Jiu (Golden Phoenix Liquor)
Ren Shen Lu Rong Wan (Ginseng and Deer Antler Pills)
Gui Zhi Jia Long Gu Mu Li Tang (Decoction of Cinnamon Twig)

Patent Formulas

Chuan Yao Tonic Pills (Strengthen Lower Back,
Make Strong Kidney Tablets)
Chin So Ku Ching—Golden Lock Tea (Golden Lock
Consolidate Jing Pills)

Jin Feng Jiu

GOLDEN PHOENIX LIQUOR

The herbs in this formula are made into a medicinal wine and used for Taoist sexual yoga and meditation. Some ingredients in it heighten sexual reproductive energies by increasing the number of sperm, and are assisted by other ingredients that are calming in an effort to lessen the tendency to spend the semen through sexual intercourse. These efforts to retain sperm are based on Taoist precepts that suggest that by conserving the seminal fluid and circulating it, abundant health, longevity, and spiritual development are advanced.

The formula Jin Feng Jiu is most effective when used while practicing sexual abstinence. It increases the vital essence (sexual reproductive energy) and quiets restlessness.

Herbal Ingredients

GRAMS NEEDED	CHINESE NAME	ENGLISH TRANSLATION
3	Sheng Di Huang	Chinese foxglove root
3	Shu Di Huang	wine-cooked Chinese foxglove root
3	Dang Gui	tang-kuei root
3	Mai Men Dong	lush winter wheat tuber
3	Di Gu Pi	wolfberry root
3	Yin Yang Huo	licentious goat wort
1.5	Sha Ren	granis of paradise

Analysis of the Herbs in This Formula

Sheng Di Huang cools the blood, and Shu Di Huang nourishes it. Dang Gui also nourishes the blood while Mai Men Dong nourishes the essence (sexual function) by increasing the production of semen. Di Gu Pi cools the interior. Yin Yang Huo strengthens sexual functioning. Sha Ren strengthens the spleen and stomach. The objective of this formula is to stimulate sexual energy and seminal production while cooling and sedating the body so that it can be conserved.

Recommended Method of Preparation
You can grind the herbs into a powder or use them whole to make
a medicinal wine. (See chapter 1 for instructions.)

Recommended Dosage
Drink 2¹/₂ to 4 ounces of Jin Feng Jiu daily at room temperature for
100 days.

REN SHEN LU RONG WAN

GINSENG AND DEER ANTLER PILLS

This formula will powerfully invigorate the chi, the jing (sexual essence), and the blood. It is extremely potent for building up and then storing energy in the Dan Tien (the body's central storage point of chi). It should be used while retaining the sexual essence.

Herbal Ingredients

GRAMS NEEDED	CHINESE NAME	ENGLISH TRANSLATION
7	Lu Rong	deer antler
6	Shan Zhu Yu	dried cornelian cherry
6	Ren Shen	ginseng root
6	Sheng Di Huang	Chinese foxglove root
6	Dang Gui	tang-kuei root
2	Rou Gui	cinnamon bark
1.5	Chen Xiang	aloeswood
1.5	Wu Wei Zi	schizandra fruit
.1	She Xiang	deer gland secretions

Analysis of the Herbs in This Formula

Lu Rong strengthens sinews and bones as well as increasing testosterone levels. Shan Zhu Yu strengthens the liver, spleen, and kidneys. Ren Shen increases chi. Sheng Di Huang cools the blood, and Dang Gui nourishes it. Rou Gui and Wu Wei Zi both nourish and restrain the essence (sexual function). Chen Xiang increases vital energy and She Xiang circulates the blood. This formula increases sexual energy, but it also includes herbs that will restrain the sperm.

Recommended Method of Preparation

Grind the herbs into a fine powder and prepare bean-sized pills. (See chapter 1 for instructions.) Traditionally, this formula was prepared as pills; if you prefer, however, you may prepare the herbs in capsule form.

Recommended Dosage

Take 1 pill or capsule daily with tepid water for 100 days.

Gui Zhi Jia Long Gu Mu Li Tang

DECOCTION OF CINNAMON TWIG

This formula restrains the essence and suppresses overstimulation and sexual dreams while regulating and harmonizing the yin and yang. It can be used by both sexes but has been found to be particularly valuable to female martial artists.

Gui Zhi Jia Long Gu Mu Li Tang meets the challenge of harmonizing sexual energies by nourishing them without overstimulating—an ongoing concern with formulas that are recommended for use in Taoist sexual practices. While excess sexual activity is believed to be a major source of energy loss, dreaming or mental preoccupation is thought to undermine concentration and mental focus. Some of the previous formulas, which are specific for sperm development, are not considered as appropriate for female martial artists as Gui Zhi Jia Long Gu Mu Li Tang. This formula contains ingredients that calm the spirit and prevent leakage of fluids yet work subtly—a quality that is generally more characteristic of the female sexual nature.

Herbal Ingredients

GRAMS NEEDED	CHINESE NAME	ENGLISH TRANSLATION
9	Gui Zhi	Saigon cinnamon twig
9	Bai Shao Yao	white peony
9	Long Gu	dragon bone
9	Sheng Jiang	ginger rhizome
9	Mu Li	oyster shell
6	Gan Cao	licorice root

PLUS

12 pieces Da Zao (jujube fruit)

Analysis of the Herbs in This Formula

Gui Zhi promotes circulation of the blood, while Bai Shao Yao and Da Zao nourish it. Long Gu and Mu Li sedate, tranquilize, and subdue hyperactivity. Sheng Jiang calms the stomach and spleen.

Gan Cao harmonizes and improves the flavor of the herbs in this formula.

Recommended Method of Preparation
Prepare a decoction. (See chapter 1 for instructions.)

Recommended Dosage
Drink 4 ounces of decocted tea at room temperature once daily. This formula should be taken for 3 to 4 days, then discontinued. You can repeat this procedure several times during a 100-day period of sexual abstinence.

Chuan Yao Tonic Pills Patent Formula

STRENGTHEN LOWER BACK, MAKE STRONG KIDNEY
TABLETS
ALSO KNOWN AS TABELLAE CHUANG YAO TONIC;
HUANG YAO JIAN SHEN PIAN

This patent medicine is very useful for replenishing jing and chi that have been lost due to sexual overindulgence. Chuan Yao Tonic Pills come in bottles of 100 or 120 pills complete with instructions on dosage. Take for 100 days.

Chin So Ku Ching—Golden Lock Tea

GOLDEN LOCK CONSOLIDATE JING PILLS
ALSO KNOWN AS JIN SUO GU JING WAN

This patent medicine will nourish the chi and astringe seminal discharge. It is extremely useful for the ejaculation control required in Taoist sexual practices. Chin So Ku Ching—Golden Lock Tea comes in bottles of 120 pills, complete with instruction on dosage. Take for 100 days.

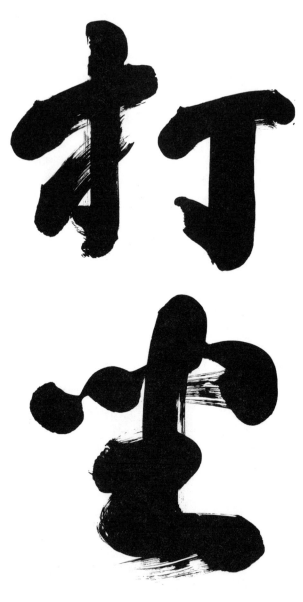

DA ZUO

MEDITATION

5

HERBS USED IN MEDITATION FOR QUIETING THE SENSES

One of the benefits of my twenty-year study of the martial arts, traditional Chinese medicine (acupuncture and herbology), Taoist esoteric yoga, and Rosicrucian philosophy has been exposure to many different forms of meditation. I have always found it interesting how little it really matters whether this activity is called meditation or prayer. In all faiths (Buddhist, Christian, Hindu, and so forth) the objective is the same—the creation of a union between the meditator and Omnipotence (God).

Beyond minor differences such as posture (Eastern crossed-leg sitting versus Western kneeling) and the use of mantras or chanting, which is mainly a feature of Eastern religions, all styles of meditation appear to be fundamentally the same. Their common objective is communication with God.

To accomplish this, three things are required:

• Quieting the mind
• Regulating the breath
• Subordinating the senses

Learning to perform slow, regulated breathing can be fairly easy. What is more difficult is developing the ability to subordinate the senses and quiet the mind.

Subordinating the senses, which means shutting out all external stimuli (sound, sight, touch, smell, and so on), is usually accomplished by retiring to a quiet, peaceful environment. Quieting the mind refers to focus—the ability to concentrate on one thing without allowing the mind to wander. An example is reciting a mantra uninterrupted for a period of time.

This is not a how-to book on meditation, of course, so I will not delve further into details explaining the process. At this point you are probably wondering how all this relates to martial arts and herbology! Well, let me explain. According to historical accounts the Chinese martial arts can be traced back to the legendary Shaolin Temple (Monastery). It was there that monks established a relationship between meditation and the martial arts.

We are told that meditation was at the center of monastic life, and that the development of martial arts (combat skills) was secondary to the monks' main purpose—spiritual development.

The spiritual development that is enhanced by regular meditation is important to the martial artists for several reasons:

- For mitigating aggressive tendencies that can develop as a result of practicing martial arts
- As an antidote to fear, which is a normal response to the threat of bodily harm during combat
- For developing an increased level of concentration and focus, which is useful during combat

It is well recognized that the development of these psychic skills is one of the most important criteria distinguishing advanced martial artists from those of lesser skill.

An integral part of the monk–martial artist lifestyle was the use of herbs. In addition to curing illness and maintaining good health, certain herbal formulas were found to be useful aids for meditation. These formulas contained herbs known to calm the *shen* (Chinese for "mind-spirit") and abate restlessness. The calming effects of these formulas created a deeper state of relaxation, thereby intensifying meditation.

This chapter contains formulas used by monks in connection with meditation and religious ceremonies. They can be useful in your efforts to achieve deeper states of relaxation and meditation.

Herbal Formulas Used as Meditation Aids to Quiet the Senses and Abate Restlessness

Raw Form Preparations

Er Miao An Shen Tang (Two-Herb Formula for Calming the Spirit)
An Shen Jing Nao Fang (Calm the Spirit and Tranquilize the Mind Formula)

Patent Formula

An Mien Pien (Peaceful Sleep Tablets)

Er Miao An Shen Tang
TWO-HERB FORMULA FOR CALMING THE SPIRIT

Although Er Miao An Shen Tang contains only two ingredients, they are both specific for calming the spirit, tranquilizing the mind, and abating restlessness and irritability. Their synergistic interaction causes each to increase or strengthen the function of the other. While this formula will not cause you to become drowsy or stupefied, its effects will be noticeable—and I recommend its use during meditation.

Herbal Ingredients

GRAMS NEEDED	CHINESE NAME	ENGLISH TRANSLATION
15	Long Gu	dragon bone
9	Suan Zao Ren	sour jujube seed

Analysis of the Herbs in This Formula
Long Gu settles and calms the spirit; it is used to abate restlessness and subdue agitation. Suan Zao Ren calms the spirit and cures irritability.

Recommended Method of Preparation
Simmer the herb Long Gu for 20 minutes before adding the Suan Zao Ren. Then prepare a decoction using the standard directions (see chapter 1).

Recommended Dosage
Drink 4 ounces of decoction at room temperature daily. Because this formula calms the spirit and abates restlessness, it is tradition-ally used ceremonially or when you are embarking on deep meditation. You can therefore use it as needed.

AN SHEN JING NAO FANG

CALM THE SPIRIT AND TRANQUILIZE THE MIND FORMULA

The qualities of certain formulas have a greater appeal to some of us, for any number of reasons. This is not to say that one is better than another; the preference is sometimes based on taste or simply on the way that a particular formula makes us feel. The effects of An Shen Jing Nao Fang are similar to and conceivably a bit milder than the last formula's. You might try it, too, for enhancing meditation.

The herbs in it should be ground into a fine powder and stored in a bottle. Take a small amount of the prepared herb mixture daily with a mixture of half water and half sweet rice wine.

Herbal Ingredients

GRAMS NEEDED	CHINESE NAME	ENGLISH TRANSLATION
9	Fu Shen	tuckahoe spirit fungus
9	Yi Zhi Ren	benefit intelligence nut
.3	Zhen Zhu	pearl
.3	Ping Sha	borax
.6	Hu Po	amber
.6	Zhu Sha	cinnabar
1.5	Mu Xiang	costus root

Analysis of the Herbs in This Formula

The herbs Fu Shen, Zhen Zhu, and Hu Po all sedate, pacify the spirit, and tranquilize. Zhu Sha also has a mild sedative effect. Mu Xiang promotes the flow of chi, and Ping Sha clears heat. Yi Zhi Ren benefits the spleen and kidney while it mitigates the harsh effects of the other herbs in this formula.

Recommended Method of Preparation

Grind the herbs into a powder and store for later use in a glass container.

Recommended Dosage

Mix .06 gram of powder with 2 ounces of sweet rice wine and 2 ounces of tepid water. Drink 3 times daily. Because this formula calms the spirit and abates restlessness, it is traditionally used ceremonially or when you are embarking on deep meditation. You can therefore use it as needed.

An Mien Pien
Patent Formula

PEACEFUL SLEEP TABLETS

ALSO KNOWN AS AN MIAN PIAN

This patent medicine will calm the spirit and tranquilize the mind. An Mien Pien comes in boxes of 60 tablets, complete with instructions on dosage.

6 In Closing

The information I have offered you in this book is based on five thousand years of Chinese herbal tradition. It is my opinion that the importance and effectiveness of using herbs in the practice of martial arts have been validated by this continuous use. And while I do agree that the martial arts have to some extent benefited from some of the nontraditional concepts that are the basis for many of the new teaching and training methods, I also feel that with modernization has come a gradual loss of some of the martial arts' traditional elements.

Among the notable casualties has been the relationship between herbology and the martial arts. Although many modernists continue to emphasize the principles of health and nutrition promoted by traditionalists in relationship to training and physical conditioning, there is also a current tendency to substitute vitamin pills and powdered protein supplements for herbal tonics and training formulas. I am also convinced that the omission of herbal use, along with other aesthetic elements, from martial arts training has contributed to the contemporary preoccupation with teaching fighting techniques at the expense of spiritual nurturing.

Still, traditionalists should not assume that the ideas I have expressed are a condemnation of all the methods currently used in martial arts training. While some are indeed questionable, others have proved their effectiveness. My intention is not to advocate the exclusion of all modern methods as much as it is to encourage the inclusion of traditional ones.

I am convinced that the future of martial arts will depend on the ability of the new breed of martial artist to integrate modern methods with traditional concepts, thereby reestablishing lost aesthetics while restoring a measure of the respect to which all forms of martial arts are entitled.

In the years ahead it will be interesting to see whether the martial arts join other forms of athletics by adopting Western sports medicine as its primary therapy, or whether practitioners will return to the use of Chinese herbal medicine that has endured for so many centuries.

APPENDIX 1

RAW HERBAL FORMULAS INDEX

Appendix 2

Patent Formulas Index

Appendix 3

Chinese Herbs Cross-Referenced to Scientific and English Names

CHINESE NAME	SCIENTIFIC NAME	ENGLISH NAME
Bai Dou Kou	*Amomum compactum*	cardamom
Bai Fu Zi	*Typhonii gigantei* rhizoma	white appendage rhizome
Bai Ji	*Bletilla striata*	bletilla rhizome
Bai Shao	*Paeonia lactiflora*	white peony root
Bai Shao Yao	*Paeonia lactiflora*	white peony
Bai Shuang	*Pulvis fumi carbonisati*	fumaria dust
Bai Zhi	*Angelica* spp.	angelica root
Bai Zhu	*Atractylodes macrocephala*	atractylodis rhizome
Ban Xia	*Pinelliae ternatae* rhizoma	half summer
Bi Ba	*Piper sylvaticum*	long pepper fruit
Bing Pian	*Cinnamomum camphora*	camphor resin
Bo He	*Mentha x piperita*	peppermint
Bu Gu Zhi	*Psoralea coryliflorliae*	scuffy pea fruit
Che Qian Zi	*Plantago asiatica*	plantago seed
Chen Pi	*Citrus reticulata*	ripe tangerine peel
Chen Xiang	*Aquilaria agallocha*	aloeswood

CHINESE NAME	SCIENTIFIC NAME	ENGLISH NAME
Chi Shao	*Paeonia veitchii*	red peony
Chuan Wu Tou	*Aconitum* spp.	processed aconite appendage
Chuan Xiong	*Ligusticum wallichii*	lovage root
Da Huang	*Rheum palmatum*	rhubarb root
Da Zao	*Ziziphus jujuba*	jujube fruit
Dang Gui	*Angelica sinensis*	tang-kuei root
Dang Shen	*Codoonopsis pilosula*	relative root
Deer Antler	(See Lu Rong)	
Deer Antler Glue	(See Lu Jiao Jiao)	
Di Gu Pi	*Lycium chinensis*	wolfberry root
Ding Xiang	*Syzygium aromaticum*	clove flower bud
Du Zhong	*Eucommia ulmoides*	eucommia bark
E Jiao	*Asini* gelatinum	donkey skin glue
Er Cha	*Acacia catechu*	cutch paste
Fang Feng	*Ledebouriellae sesloidis* radix	guard against wind
Feng Xian Hua	*Impatiens balsamina*	impatiens flower
Fu Ling	*Poria cocos*	tuckahoe root
Fu Pen Zi	*Rubus chingii*	Chinese raspberry fruit
Fu Shen	*Poria cocos pararadicis Scolerotuim*	tuckahoe spirit fungus
Fu Zi	*Aconitum carmichaelii*	aconite root
Gan Cao	*Glycyrrhiza uralensis*	licorice root
Ge Jie	*Gekko gecko*	gecko lizard
Ginger	(See Sheng Jiang)	
Ginseng Root	(See Ren Shen)	
Gou Gu	*Canine* os	dog bone
Gou Qi Zi	*Lycium barbarum*	matrimony fruit
Gua Lou	*Trichosanthes kirilowii*	heavenly flower fruit
Gui Zhi	*Cinnamomum cassia*	Saigon cinnamon twig
Gu Sui Bu	*Gusuibu* rhizoma	mender of shattered bones rhizome
Hai Ma	*Hippocampus* spp.	sea horse
Hei Jing Jie	*Schizonepetae tenuifoliae* flos	blackened jingjie

CHINESE NAME	SCIENTIFIC NAME	ENGLISH NAME
Hong Hua	*Carthamus tinctorius*	safflower
Huang Bai	*Phellodendron amurense*	cork tree bark
Huang Lian	*Coptis chinense*	golden thread
Huang Qi	*Astragalus membranaceus*	milk vetch root
Hu Gu	*Tigris os*	tiger bone*
Hu Po	*Succinum*	amber
Jiang Huang	*Curcuma domestica*	turmeric rhizome
Jie Geng	*Platycodon grandiflorum*	balloonflower root
Jin Yin Hua	*Lonicera japonica*	honeysuckle flower
Ji Xue Teng	*Millettia reticulata*	chicken blood vine
Liu Ji Nu	*Artemisiae anomalae* herba	Liu's residing slave
Long Gu	*Draconis os*	dragon bone
Lu Jiao Jiao	*Cervus nippon temminck*	deer antler glue
Lu Rong	*Cervus nippon*	deer antler
Ma Bo	*Lasiophaera fenslii*	puffball fruit
Ma Qian Zi	*Strychnos nux-vomica*	nux vomica seed
Ma Huang	*Ephedra minima*	hemp yellow
Mai Men Dong	*Ophiogon japonicus*	lush winter wheat tuber
Ming Tian Ma	*Gastrodiae elatae* rhizoma	heavenly hemp
Mo Yao	*Commiphora myrrah*	myrrh
Mu Dan Pi	*Paeonia suffruticosa*	peony root bark
Mu Gua	*Chaenomeles speciosa*	quince fruit
Mu Li	*Concha ostreae*	oyster shell
Mu Tong	*Mutong caulis*	wood with holes
Mu Xiang	*Saussureae sen vladimiriae*	costus root
Nan Xing	*Arisaema triphyllum*	jack in the pulpit rhizome
Niu Xi	*Achyranthes bidentata*	ox-knee root
Nu Zhen Zi	*Ligustrum lucidum*	privet fruit
Peng Sha or Ping Sha	*Borax*	borax
Qing Pi	*Citrus reticulata*	green tangerine peel

*Tiger bone is an illegal substance inthe United States. See pages 77–78 for more on this subject.

CHINESE NAME	SCIENTIFIC NAME	ENGLISH NAME
Ren Shen	*Panax ginseng*	ginseng root
Rou Gui	*Cinnamomum cassia*	cinnamon bark
Ru Xiang	*Boswellia carterii*	frankincense
Sha Ren	*Amomi fructus seu* semen	grains of paradise seed
Shan Zhu Yu	*Cornus officinalis*	dried cornelian cherry
Shan Yao	*Dioscorea opposita*	Chinese yam root
She Xiang	*Moschus moschiferus*	deer gland secretions
Sheng Di Huang	*Rehmannia glutinosa*	Chinese foxglove root
Sheng Jiang	*Zingiber officinale*	ginger rhizome
Shu Di Huang	*Rehmannia glutinosa*	wine-cooked Chinese foxglove root
Suan Zao Ren	*Ziziphus jujuba* var. *spinosa*	sour jujube seed
Suo Yang	*Cynomorium songaricum*	lock yang stem
Tao Ren	*Persicae semen*	peach pit kernel
Tian Chi Ginseng	*Panax pseudoginseng*	pseudo ginseng root
Tiger Bone	(See Hu Gu)	
Tu Bie Chong	*Eupolyhaga sinensis*	wingless cockroach
Tu Si Zi	*Cuscutae* semen	dodder seed
Wu Jia Pi	*Eleutherococcus gracilistylis*	five-bark root
Wu Wei Zi	*Schisandra chinensis*	schizandra fruit
Xiang Fu	*Cyperus rotundus*	nut grass rhizome
Xiao Hui Xiang	*Foeniculum vulgare*	fennel fruit
Xu Duan	*Dipsacus japonica*	teasel root
Xue Jie	*Daemonorops draco*	dragon's blood resin
Xue Yu Tan	*Crinis carbonisatus*	charred human hair
Yang Ti	*Capra*	goat hooves
Ye Ju Hua	*Chrysanthemum indicum*	chrysanthemum flower
Yi Zhi Ren	*Alpiniae oxphyllae* fructus	benefit intelligence nut
Yin Yang Huo	*Epimedii herba licentious*	licentious goat wort
Yu Jin	*Curcuma longa*	turmeric tuber
Ze Xie	*Alisma plantago-aquatica*	water plantain
Zhang Nao	*Cinnamomum camphora*	camphor
Zhen Zhu	*Pteria magaritifera*	pearl

CHINESE NAME	SCIENTIFIC NAME	ENGLISH NAME
Zhi Qiao	*Citri seu ponciri* immaturus	bitter orange fruit
Zhi Zi	*Gardenia jasminoides*	gardenia fruit
Zhu Gan Cao	*Glycyrrhiza uralensis*	honey-cooked licorice
Zhu Sha	*Cinnabaris*	cinnabar
Zi He Che	*Hominis* placenta	human placenta
Zi Ran Tong or Zi Ran Ton	*Pyritum*	pyrite
Zi Su Ye	*Perilla frutescens*	perilla leaf

Appendix 4

Sources for Herbal and Patent Formulas

The following companies specialize in mail-order sales of herbs and herbal formulas and will supply you with a mail-order catalog on request.

To purchase herbs in bulk, patent formulas, or any of the herbal formulas discussed in this book, contact:

Treasures from the Sea of Chi
360 Grand Street, Suite 124
Oakland, CA 94610
Phone: 510-451-7470
Fax: 510-452-3550
E-mail: TJSeaOfChi@AOL.com

To purchase herbs in bulk or patent formulas:

Mayway Trading Company
1338 Cypress Street
Oakland, CA 94607
Phone: 510-208-3123

Chinese patent medicines may be purchased from the following Chinese herb stores from throughout the United States. All of these companies have employees who speak English:

BAC-A1 Pharmacy
216B Canal Street
New York, NY 10013
Phone: 212-513-1344

North South China Herb Company
1556 Stockton Street
San Francisco, CA 94134
Phone: 415-421-4907

Wing Fung Tai Ginseng Company
833 North Broadway
Los Angeles, CA 90012
Phone: 213-617-0699

Essential Chinese Herb Store
646 North Spring Street
Los Angeles, CA 90012
Phone: 213-680-1374

Golden Import
46 Beach Street
Boston, MA 02111
Phone: 617-350-7001

Cheng Kwong Market
73–79 Essex Street
Boston, MA 02111
Phone: 617-482-3221

Vinh Kan Ginseng Company
675 Washington Street
Boston, MA 02111
Phone: 617-338-9028

The following are mail-order herb companies that sell a wide variety of Western and Chinese herbs. Call for one of their catalogs or to place an order over the phone. All have employees who speak English.

Penn Herb Company
10601 Decatur Road, #2
Philadelphia, PA 19154
Phone: 1-800-523-9971

Nuherbs
3820 Penniman Avenue
Oakland, CA 94510
Phone: 510-534-HERB

Kwok Shing Import Export Inc.
1818 Harrison Street
San Francisco, CA 94103
Phone: 415-861-1668

APPENDIX 5

REFERENCE SOURCES FOR HERBAL FORMULAS

Dan Bensky, *Chinese Herbal Medicine Materia Medica* (Seattle, Wash.: Eastland Press, 1990).

Bob Flaws, *Chinese Medicine in Injury Management* (Boulder, Colo.: Blue Poppy Press, 1983).

Bob Flaws, *Secret Formulas for the Treatment of External Injury* (Boulder, Colo.: Blue Poppy Press, 1995).

Jake Fratkin, *Chinese Herbal Patent Formulas* (Boulder, Colo.: Shya Publications, 1986).

James Ramholz, *Shaolin and Taoist Herbal Formulas* (Chicago: Silk Road, 1992).

Echoes From Old China (Honolulu, Hawaii: University Of Hawaii Press, 1989).

Chinese Herbal: An Introduction (Honolulu, Hawaii: Tai School of Philosophy and Art, 1982).